THE HONEY BOOK

By Emily Thacker

Published by:

James Direct Inc

500 S. Prospect Ave.

Hartville, Ohio 44632

U.S.A.

ISBN: 978-1-62397-048-2

Printing 12 11 10 9 8 7 6 5 4 3 2

First Edition   **Copyright 2012**   **James Direct Inc**

TABLE OF CONTENTS

A Letter from Emily

Dear Reader,

It is with much anticipation and pleasure that I bring to you, *The Honey Book*, the latest in my series of natural home health books. I want to personally thank you for your continued interest in this series of books aimed at making for a healthier life, and getting there the natural way. The enthusiasm shared in your letters is a constant source of encouragement to me, and much of the reason for bringing you this new book.

We are all familiar with honey as that sticky staple in our home pantry we throw on the top of a stack of pancakes or use as that special ice cream topping. Honey can be found in numerous gourmet baking recipes including a ham or pork chop glaze, or fancy homemade nougats and candies. (By the way, be sure and reference the special recipe chapter near the back of this book for fantastic ways to incorporate honey into your daily diet.)

But, while past generations touted honey as a must-have staple in every home, it was for a very different reason. It was understood that honey possessed special qualities that made it the treatment of choice for everyday health conditions and maladies that ailed the human body. Our elders found that, for whatever reason, honey was helpful in treating cuts and open sores, and used to promote healing in burns and scalds. It was taken orally to gently soothe an upset stomach or as a quick fix for gastritic issues. Honey was commonly used for colds and sore throats.

For centuries, honey has been used as not only as a remedy for countless ailments and health conditions, but also for its benefits as an external healing salve. Honey has been used as a wound dressing for soldiers on the battlefield. Honey has can be found as a main ingredient in many herb-based home remedies for treating every condition from asthma and tuberculosis to whooping cough and bronchitis.

But just how much of this was wishful folklore, and how much has been backed up by scientific and medical research? I asked myself that very question. And the answers I found after years of research might just surprise you. *Pleasantly* surprise you!

Years of research into the effects of honey on the human body has provided the scientific community with a better understanding of its countless benefits, both consumed internally to treat common maladies, and as an external healing element.

Nutrition-wise, we have always known this sweet substance provides several types of carbohydrates for a quick energy release. But researchers have also identified 19 different proteins in just one single variety of Australian honey. It is a wonderfully fat-free food that can be helpful not only with digestive issues, but has also been known as a remedy for allergies.

In-depth studies from the research community into the health benefits of honey have been ongoing for decades. Studies from world renown research facilities, such as the famous Cairo University to publications such as the *American Journal of Surgery* have touted research sharing the surprising health benefits and healing properties of honey.

For example, did you know that honey has been used in hospitals as a surgical dressing on post-operative wounds with amazing results? Studies have also shown that honey can not only accelerate wound healing times, but may also leave behind less scar tissue as it is less likely to irritate surrounding, unaffected skin tissue than many prescribed salves.

It is currently being used as a more gentle treatment for nursing home patients suffering from painful bedsores and even being studied as a treatment for gangrene patients with much success. Physicians are using honey solutions as a way of preserving delicate skin grafts and prolonging the viability of corneas as they await transplant. Honey has been proven to contain antifungal and antibacterial properties making it an ideal dressing for many situations.

Would you believe research is showing honey to contain properties that enable some cancer fighting drugs to work more effectively?

Hence the purpose for my writing this book. To introduce you to an amazing array of uses for this wonderful, natural substance honey. A substance you can use confidently, without so many of the side effects we have come to expect from chemical-based tonics and medications.

In *The Honey Book*, you will learn about how honey is being used to treat conditions such as:

- Boosting immune systems
- Cough suppressant
- Arthritis
- Digestive problems
- Constipation
- Diarrhea
- Respiratory infections
- Sore throats
- Fever reducers
- Insomnia
- Treat cold sores
- Ease shingle pain
- Weight loss issues
- Joint pain
- Goiter
- Burns
- Bedsores

...just to name a few!

The research is exciting and fascinating – and ongoing! While we have only scratched the surface into the health benefits of honey, it is already being put to use medically worldwide. This is just the beginning! Scientists and researchers have learned some amazing properties regarding the makeup of honey that we are just beginning to understand.

We know that honey is:

- Fat free
- Cholesterol free
- Rich in antioxidants
- Contains vitamins
- Contains proteins
- Minerals
- Antifungal
- Antibacterial
- Anti inflammatory
- Antiproliferative
- Able to make some cancer-fighting drugs more effective

Its soothing properties even cross over into the world of skin and beauty aids, as it is used for everything from softening the skin to promoting luxurious hair. You'll read about some of the most ideal uses for honey as a beauty regimen, like:

- Facial scrub
- Hair conditioner
- Skin softener and toner
- Facial cleanser

- Treating acne
- Moisturizer
- Bath and shower gel

Since before recorded history, many have felt honey should be part of a wholesome diet and healthy lifestyle. Today, we know exercise and proper nutrition can help you control our medical future. For most people, this can include honey's sweet goodness. Because honey is a fat free, cholesterol free food, it has been linked to many weight loss diets and regimens.

Like many good things, honey also has a down side. Some honey has been found to carry botulinum spores that are especially dangerous to infants. Because of this warning, babies under 1 year of age SHOULD NEVER BE GIVEN HONEY.

Please note, that some of what is contained in *The Honey Book* is history. It relates the way others, in tradition, myth and even worship, have used honey. The decision as to whether or not it is useful in today's world must be left to you, the reader.

Do remember, old-time remedies have an important place in our culture, and can be very useful in a healthy lifestyle. But, they cannot take the place of medical advice. When you are sick, you should seek the advice of a competent medical practitioner. For everyday healthy living, you may want to incorporate honey into your life.

Thank you for reading.
Emily

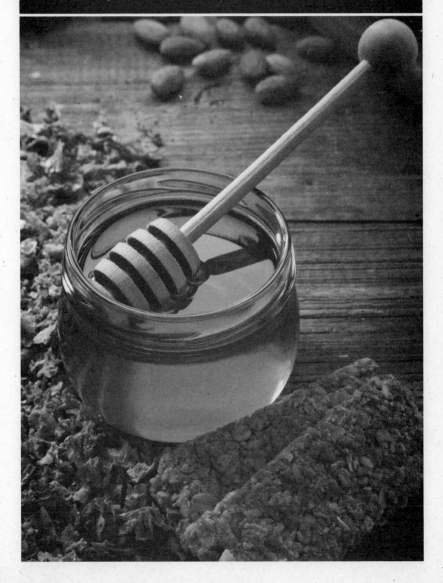

CHAPTER ONE
Introduction

We are proud to introduce to you, *The Honey Book*. *The Honey Book* is the most recent release in a series of health, remedy and natural living books written by world renowned author, Emily Thacker.

Throughout her career as natural health author, Emily has sold more than 5 million books stemming from her research into better living, the natural way. Her signature series book entitled *The Vinegar Book*, has sold more than 4 million copies worldwide. (You may wish to reference the appendices in the back of this book for descriptions of additional home, health and natural remedy books as an accompaniment to this book).

Each of Emily's books contain practical advice for living life more naturally and contain countless home and health solutions derived from everyday items that are probably staples in your own home pantry. Items such as apple cider vinegar, garlic, baking soda, hydrogen peroxide and now honey.

The Honey Book is the result of years of research and study into the effects and health benefits of honey on the human body.

So, why a book about honey?
Honey itself has been around since the beginning of time. Its history is rich, dating back centuries. It includes both pilgrims and prophets, princes and peasants. Honey has been given as dowry. It has been used to entomb the dead in burial ceremonies. Honey was sometimes considered the treasure of royalty.

Honey is a delightful food, rich in goodness. That same goodness is the preferred sweetener of choice in gourmet recipes throughout Europe. What would Mediterranean baklava be without the golden, sweet flow of honey?

However, for centuries honey has also been used as something else. It has been used as both a healing salve for cuts and open wounds and also the basis in elixirs for common ailments and maladies of the body. Honey has been commonly used in teas to soothe digestive tracts or taken by the spoonful to ease the discomfort of a sore throat. Historically, honey was used on the battlefield as a dressing for battle wounds, and on open cuts to deter infection.

While these treatments often worked, and many times were successful with amazing results, it was not always known *why* honey was beneficial to the human body. *The Honey Book* will not only explore the makeup of honey, but how to incorporate it as a home remedy staple.

Remedies for honey seem endless and there are literally countless uses for it on every day ailments. A few of its uses include:

- As a salve on baby's skin
- Soothe chapped lips
- Wrap poultices around aching joints for relief from joint pain
- Open breathing tracts
- Relief from sore throat pain
- Ease respiratory infections

- Hydrate dry mouth conditions
- Use as a natural laxative
- Treatment for indigestion
- Prevent infection in cuts and scrapes
- Lotion for rough, chapped hands
- Fights insomnia
- Treatment for sunburns
- Preventative measure for allergies
- Digestive aid

But honey is so much more – and the scientific community is conducting new research to back up some startling findings. Findings that put honey in an entirely new light.

The Honey Book hopes to bring these finding to light. *The Honey Book* traces honey throughout history, chronicling its place and rise throughout the ages. Readers will explore its origins is fact and fiction. We will look at the entire process of the bees laborious endeavor to make honey and how that directly benefits us. We will also review the old time, home remedy uses for honey and how those were a stepping stone to some of the more recent scientific findings and successes in regard to honey in the field of medicine. Some of these findings being quite amazing.

And of course, we will look at ways to incorporate honey into everyday life, whether it be through simple home remedies or course of treatments to ask your physician or health care provider about, along with recipes to bring honey into mealtime planning.

Why consider honey?

As you know, honey is a natural substance found liberally in nature. Unlike so many of the chemical-based drugs and medications being introduced into our bodies laced with chemicals and manufactured additives, honey is all-natural. While many of these medications come with series side-effects (sometimes creating a trade-off from one problem to another), honey contains none of the harmful chemicals which produce many of those unwanted additions. Today's medications come with warnings of harmful side effects, or medications that cannot safely be used in conjunction with one another. Honey does not present this problem.

And unfortunately, although many times medications or remedies that are within reach at the nearest drug store or pharmacy, they may not be easily afforded. Honey is inexpensive and easy to purchase at any grocery store. It may very well be waiting in your kitchen pantry right now.

Now, please understand what is being said, and more importantly, what is NOT being said. Not all commercially manufactured medication is bad. Quite the opposite. Many pharmaceuticals are imperative for treating numerous conditions and diseases. And sometimes chronic pain can only be alleviated through a plan laid out by your physician or health care provider.

But, if there is a better, more wholesome and natural way available, why not explore it?

The Honey Book examines one simple ingredient, and the research that goes along with it, to help provide you with an alternative when making your health care decisions.

Medicinal Uses

Honey, particularly honey that is used in its more raw form, can bear an amazing assortment of remedies and treatments when used both internally and externally.

Studies from the research community indicate that honey contains properties making it ideal as a natural healing remedy. The scientific compositional breakdown of honey confirms what other generations seemed to know instinctively: honey for medicinal uses is not just idle folklore. There is real science behind the healing attributes of honey.

As will be explained in greater detail in later chapters, honey contains elements which make it both antibacterial (meaning that its elements actively fight bacteria) and antimicrobial (meaning that it kills or retards the growth of microbial organisms). These two aspects make it a prime source of healing for simple cuts, scrapes and abrasions. But science has actually taken honey's use a step further.

The breakdown and research into honey has revealed that the makeup of honey contains an enzyme which, when released, exudes low levels of hydrogen peroxide. This release of hydrogen peroxide makes it ideal for treating bacteria-laced wounds, as it works to kill bacteria on contact.

In the medical field, hydrogen peroxide or hydrogen peroxide derivatives and products are many times used as a bacteria-fighting element in the triage of open wounds. The problem with hydrogen peroxide is that while it works to kill bacteria and heal the open wound, it can, at the same time, be damaging to the surrounding healthy tissue. It does not differentiate between healthy and unhealthy tissue.

Honey, while still fighting bacteria with its own hydrogen peroxide solution, has been found to not damage the surrounding healthy tissue. In fact, its balm-like properties, and the fact that hydrogen peroxide is released at low levels, actually works to protect and heal surrounding tissue.

Some studies have gone on to show that patients treated with honey, versus patients treated with more conventional methods, many times indicate faster healing times and quicker recovery. Researchers also feel patients were left with less unsightly scar tissue.

But that's just the beginning. Hospitals around the world have been studying the effects of honey as a treatment with great success. Just a few of the areas of treatment achievement include:

- Gangrenous patients
- Hospital and nursing home patients with painful bedsores
- Post-operative incision healing

- Burn and scald victims
- Skin graft preservation
- Soak for cornea transplants
- Surgical dressing
- Antifungal cream
- Anti-inflammatory illnesses
- Reduce the risk of heart disease
- Improving the effectiveness of some cancer fighting medications
- Allergy preventative
- Antiproliferate agent
- Arthritic symptoms

Studies also tout honey's preventative benefits in health, particularly where heart disease is of concern. Because honey is a cholesterol free food, it can easily be substituted in the place of other sweeteners in the diet as a way of eliminating extra cholesterol in the daily menu.

Honey has also shown to not only reduce cholesterol levels in patients, but also bring down dangerous CRP levels (C-reactive protein), which many physicians believe is also an early indicator of heart disease and other serious medical conditions.

For years in Australia, "medicinal" grade honey has been used in hospitals and physicians offices as an effective treatment for open wounds. In many areas around the world, one can even purchase honey bandages. These bandages are already infused with high grade medicinal honey as their active healing element.

And studies into medical uses for honey continue in hospitals and research centers worldwide. Researchers have documented countless remedial uses for honey, and even more have been handed down through past generations.

Yet there is much more left to be discovered. *The Honey Book* hopes to introduce you to the new world of honey, and then act as a springboard for new uses of your own.

A word of caution for infants

Like most good things, honey has its downside. Many of the remedies in the book call for taking honey orally. While honey is an all-natural nutritious food, it is important to never give honey to an infant. Guidelines call for **honey to be never given to a baby under one year of age**.

This also applies to using honey as a salve for treating cuts or scrapes to babies. Because babies can be counted on to put everything in their mouth, you would not want to use honey as a salve on an open sore until the child reaches one year of age.

Consulting your health care practitioner

Remember that while many uses are very helpful today, still others may not be the best solution in today's world. Be sure and speak with your healthcare practitioner before making regular use of any home remedy, whether it is honey, hydrogen peroxide, baking soda, vinegar or any other food or substance.

It is my sincere desire that this information will act as a springboard for conversation between you and your healthcare provider, opening up additional avenues of treatment for everyday illnesses…the natural way.

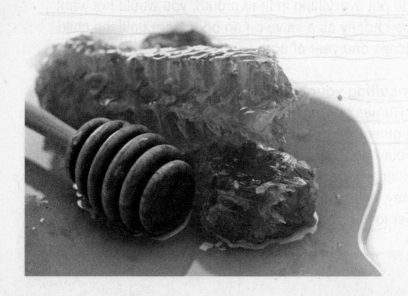

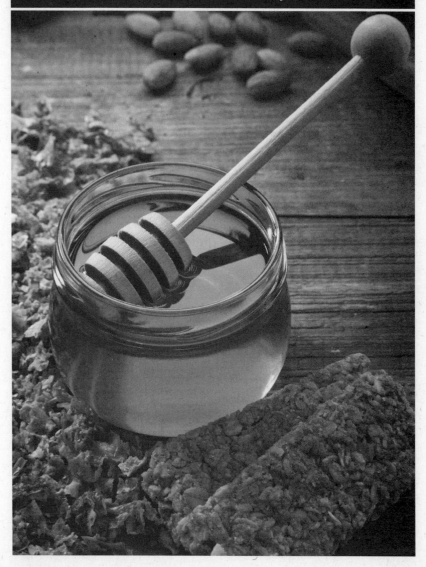

CHAPTER TWO
What is Honey?

Honey is nature's original sweetener, and unlike sugar, only a bee can make true honey. Honey can be white or pale cream in color, gold or bronze, amber or yellow. It can be brown or purple. There is even an African honey that is clear green, sealed in bright red combs.

Honey is sweet flower nectar which has had some of its water evaporated out, then wondrously changed into thick golden goodness by the work of industrious honey bees. It is actually a predigested food, so only a very small amount of energy is needed for the body to use it.

Honey is an amazing combination of substances healthy to the human body. Rich in carbohydrates, it is mostly an assortment of dissolved sugars, such as sucrose, glucose and fructose. It also contains a wide array of minerals, vitamins, pigments, enzymes and amino acids. And, good for cancer-fighting properties, honey even contains highly regarded antioxidant properties.

For the health conscious, honey is both fat free and cholesterol free. But the most important parts of honey may be the ones that have not been identified at all! The most elaborate chemical analysis cannot fully explain the amazing properties of honey -- or even identify all the various healthful substances bees and flowers put in it.

How Bees Do It
Nectar from flowers is, for the most part, made up of sucrose and water. Doing their wonderful magic, bees infuse special enzymes that when added create a unique

chemical reaction which then converts sucrose into both glucose and fructose sugars. Evaporation then occurs which removes excess water leaving behind a rich, golden honey that resists spoilage and breakdown.

So, just how exactly do bees do it?

Bees collect the thin, lightly sweetened nectar that rests in the heart of most flowers. They collect, first, from species with the highest sugar content. Sometimes they even gather sweet juice from damaged fruit.

Only a bee can change nectar into honey. Nectar is sucked up by forager bees and stored within their honey sacs. When the bees return to the hive, they spit up the nectar, which is now mixed with special digestive enzymes, and pass it on to other worker bees.

One of these enzymes, invertase, changes a complicated sugar in the nectar into two simpler sugars. As the liquid is passed from bee to bee, more enzymes are added and much of the moisture is evaporated. The mixture becomes thicker, sweeter and more concentrated.

Enzymes are complex protein-based substances that can only be made by living cells. In a nearly "magical" manner, these enzymes encourage chemical reactions, such as inversion, to take place -- often without any apparent change to themselves. Yet, these reactions only take place if some of the enzyme is present.

Inversion is the chemical term that describes how a complex sugar is divided into two (or more) simple sugars. Enzymes in honey also act as fermenting agents. They are catalysts that encourage the changes which turn thin nectar into thick, rich honey. (The enzymes in honey may also be the substance that indefinitely prolongs honey's shelf life.)

For example, one enzyme, invertase, makes saccharose (a double sugar) divide into two single sugars (dextrose and fructose). Another double sugar, sucrose, is divided into glucose and fructose.

The dividing of sugars is the beginning of the digestive process. Therefore, because honey is partially predigested, it is very easy for the human body to absorb its nutrients.

Honey is about twice as sweet as most nectar. This is because bees concentrate nectar by evaporating the water out of it.

A worker bee holds a drop of nectar on the end of its tongue, exposing it to the air. Then the bee swallows the nectar and repeats the process. After 80 or so times the nectar is both concentrated and partially digested by enzymes in the bee's body.

When the bees have finished making honey, they seal it in wax cells. Here, the invertase continues its action of acting on sugars. When the honey is completely finished, it is considered "ripe."

The invertase in honey is very sensitive to heat. If the honey is allowed to get too hot, the invertase is permanently ruined.

Yeasts thrive in honey that has a high water content. So, sometimes commercial honey packers heat the honey in a pasteurization process to destroy these potentially unhealthy yeasts. Or, they use high pressure to force heated honey through filters. This produces a clear, light colored product.

Traditionally, honey was prepared by straining broken combs, slowly, through a cloth bag. Any cold-process honey has a more natural flavor than one extracted with heat.

When honey is heated, some of the aromatic oils from flower blossom nectar are released. Too much heat can leave honey bland and tasteless.

Usually, honey from a local beekeeper will be more flavorful than one that has been commercially processed. And, it may be a healthier product since, generally, it has had less processing done to it.

Sometimes Less is More

When there are fewer flower blossoms, bees must work longer and harder to collect the nectar they need. Honey made during these lean times almost always contains more beneficial bee enzymes than honey produced when nectar is plentiful.

Any nectar that is very thin and diluted needs much more processing by bees to concentrate it into honey. So, this honey will also contain more bee produced enzymes than honey made from richer, thicker, more concentrated kinds of nectars.

Honey is Concentrated Flower Power

Nearly 200 different substances have been identified in honey. Yet, examinations of honey still leave part of it as unknown or undetermined. And, no two honeys are ever exactly the same.

The weather, the kind of plants the bees visit, even the soil the flowers that supplied the nectar grew in can influence the vitamin and mineral content of honey. They will also make a difference in its color, flavor and consistency.

While most of honey is water and sugar, about 3% of it is made up of other substances. These can be vitamins, pigments, enzymes, hormones from plants, organic acids, minerals, amino acids, or other proteins.

And, there are nearly 50 types of aromatic substances in honey, although only about two dozen have been fully identified.

Honey can sometimes host additional particles or artifacts floating within its goodness. Natural honey can contain small pieces of dead bees, comb fragments, grains of sand, bee hairs and pollen grains. Some of these particles, such as pollen grains or spores, are actually beneficial. As we will discuss in greater detail in a later chapter, pollen trapped from local sources has been shown to help relieve allergy symptoms with an immunizing effect.

Each batch of honey, even if it is from the same bees and the same hive, varies in color, flavor, aroma, texture, enzymes, vitamins and mineral content.

Some general acids that can be found in honey include:
/5
- Acetic
- Malic
- Benzoic
- Oxalic
- Butyric
- Phenylacetic
- Citric
- Propionic
- Formic
- Gluconic
- Pyroglutamic
- Isovaleric
- Succinic
- Lactic
- Valeric

Most of the amino acids which are found in honey are derived from the pollen grains that have been mixed in with the honey. Amino acids are breakdowns of more complex proteins. They can be used to help to differentiate which honey is which, and to identify which might be adulterated with fillers.

Some amino acids that can be found in honey are:

16

- Aspartic acid
- Isoleucine
- Alanine
- Methionine
- Arginine
- Phenylalanine
- Cystine
- Proline
- Glycine
- Serine
- Glutamic acid
- Tryptophan
- Histidine
- Tyrosine
- Lysine
- Valine

Often, in addition to pollen grains, honey has wild yeasts, algae and molds from honeydew mixed into it. Most of the vitamins in honey are concentrated within the occasional grains of pollen that may be found floating in it. Vitamin content also varies by kind of honey. For example, vitamin C is more likely to be found in citrus honeys. Not only does each honey source brings its own addition of vitamins to the final honey, but so does the actual soil in the area.

Some vitamins that can be found in honey are:

- B-1 (thiamine)
- B-2 (riboflavin)
- Nicotinic acid (niacin)
- B-6 (pyridoxine & pantothenic acid)
- C (ascorbic acid)
- K

Minerals

Generally, the darker the honey, the more minerals that are contained in it. The part of honey that contains minerals is usually referred to as its "ash content." It averages from 1% to 3% of the total weight of honey.

The tiny "ash content" part of honey packs a nutritional wallop! So far, at least 28 different minerals have been isolated in honeys.

Honey can contain many minerals, a few of which include:

- Calcium
- Copper
- Iron
- Magnesium
- Manganese
- Phosphate
- Phosphorus
- Potassium
- Silica

29

Before modern methods of geological testing were widespread, miners would sometimes analyze the mineral content of the honey in an area. This often gave the miners important clues as to the kinds of minerals that could be found in the soil.

Generally, ling, heather and honeydew honeys have a greater amount of minerals in them. Lime, sweet chestnut and mint honeys may have calcium.

Pine honey is high in iron, heather in copper, acacia in manganese. Potassium and iron can be found in all kinds of honeys.

Researchers are finding that glucose, like that in honey, can encourage the body to do a better job of absorbing minerals such as zinc and magnesium.

Honey consumption, like all good things, should not be overdone. Some new research indicates that taking in too much of such sugary substances may block calcium absorption in the intestines. Over a long period of time this could be harmful to bone growth.

Honey Can Kill Germs
The substances in honey that hold down the growth of bacteria are called inhibines. They are, mostly, by-products of glucose oxidase, an enzyme bees add to nectar when making honey.

The glucose oxidase in honey is a fermenting agent. It originates from fungus (much like penicillin does). When honey is eaten, the acid it produces is one of the things that helps the kidneys remove poisons from the body.

Glucose oxidase acts on glucose in unripened honey. It makes gluconic acid and hydrogen peroxide, which are both sensitive to light and heat. This is one reason why the best honey is never exposed to great heat or strong sunlight.

Because honey contains germ killing substances from bees, it has long been used as a sterile dressing for wounds. It also has other advantages for helping healing -- it does not dry out like most salves and it does not produce any side effects in healthy tissue.

Some researchers say the vitamin K in honey acts against the bacteria that causes tooth decay. If this proves to be true it could be one of the safest sweeteners ever!

Often, honey is added to herbal remedies. It serves to make bitter herbs taste better, and it also adds its own ability to heal.

Because of all their bacteria killing substances, many of which are just now being isolated and understood by scientists, honey, vinegar and garlic have long been an important part of folk healing remedies.

The combinations of honey and vinegar, or honey and garlic, are traditional remedies for those suffering from asthma, tuberculosis, whooping cough and bronchitis.

Tradition says that for the most effective relief of these kinds of illnesses, the best honey to eat is that of your local area. Some believe this is because of the unique pollen content of each batch of honey.

Burns

Honey has been long used as a sterile salve for burns. Because it is able to take up water from the air, it promotes healing by keeping the burns moist and not allowing tissue to dry up prematurely. It may also be able to reduce scaring because burns that are kept moist are less likely to form scabs and scar.

A Word of Caution

It is possible for honey -- particularly if it has been improperly processed or if it is very old -- to become contaminated by bacteria. This honey could be dangerous to use on burns or other open wounds.

Honeydew Honey

"Honeydew" is the thin, sweet fluid left behind on plants that have been attacked by aphids, scales or other insects. These tiny creatures live by sucking the juices of plants.

As these sucking insects feed on plant sap, they excrete the sweet-sticky substance known as honeydew. It is sometimes gathered by bees, particularly if flower nectar is scarce.

Honey from honeydew is a bit different than that made from flower nectar. In addition to the traditional honey sugars, it has enzymes from the digestive system of the insects that deposited the honeydew.

Honeydew honey contains more nitrogen, in the form of amino acids and amides, than that of nectar honey. It also has more citric acid. Depending on the conditions under which it was produced, this honey can also contain sugar alcohols such as dulcitol, sorbitol, inositol or ribitol.

In ancient times it was believed plant leaves made honeydew and then aphids came to feed on it. Science has since disproved the idea.

Granulated Honey

Honey is supersaturated with sugars. Because it is supersaturated, it will crystallize easily. Cold temperature and stirring can begin the process. Glucose is less soluble than other sugars, so granulation is more likely to occur in honey that has a high percent of glucose.

Honey that has a high percentage of other kinds of sugar (such as fructose) rarely crystallizes.

For granulation to begin there must be something in the honey for the crystals to gather onto. This can be dust particles, pollen grains, air bubbles or even the walls of the honey container.

Since dark honey usually contains more added particles than light honey, it usually crystallizes sooner. Honey that is free from particles and air bubbles, generally, will not crystallize for years.

As honey crystallizes it becomes lighter in color. So, even a dark honey tends to be light after granulation.

In Europe, most honey is served as a granulated product. Europeans prefer this and use it as a spread. In the United State, granulated honey is often considered spoiled, although this is untrue. Granulated honey is still perfectly fine for consumption. It is simply in the process of altering form from a liquid to a more solid state.

Honey which has begun to crystallize can be returned to its liquid state by warming it over the stove. If it is heated to 140° or 150°, then held there for about half an hour, most honey will not crystallize again easily. This much gentle heat does little to hurt the flavor or nutritive content. But honey should not be heated to a much higher degree.

One can also reconstitute crystallized honey by placing the affected honey jar in a pan of warm water, allowing the honey to reliquify gradually. As the honey crystals begin to dissipate, gently swirl the jar to mix together.

The crystallization process itself is much more destructive to the flavor of honey. Many honeys have a delicate fragrance that is from aromatic flower oils. These oils are very volatile.

Granulated honey has lost most of these light fragrances. For example, both thyme and marjoram honeys are known for their fine flavors. Once they have crystallized they become bland and almost tasteless.

Darker colored honeys are more apt to be highly flavored by minerals and protein containing pollen. They are much better candidates for crystallization. Ragwort and buckwheat honeys, for example, are considered by many to have flavors that are too strong for many uses. But, once crystallized, they taste much like most other honeys.

Some honey is not liquid, even when fresh. These honeys are more gels than liquids. Actually, they are very special gels. Called "thixotropic" gels, these honeys are very stiff and jellylike until stirred. Then, they rapidly become thin liquids.

Hawaiian alergoba honey is one of the kinds of honey which granulates very easily. Both heather and ling honeys are more gel-like than liquid.

From the snow-white honey of Siberia, to the black honey of Brazil, the very best honey is served fresh from the hive -- still warm from the bees!

More Type of Honey

Granulated honey is just one type of honey variation from the golden liquid honey to which we are most accustomed. Honey can also be found in solid form such as dried or whipped honeys.

The following page lists a few brief descriptions of some of the more popular honey varieties:

- **Raw honey.** This is generally honey as it presents itself straight from the beehive. True raw honey has not undergone the heating process. Although the truest raw honey has not been heated, some honey is still labeled "raw" so long as the heating process has been small enough not to effect the honey's nutritional content or consistency. It may contain "artifacts" such as pollen spores or flower particles. This is the type of local honey some allergy sufferers swear by as an "immunization" as allergy season approaches.

- **Pasteurized honey**. As with milk, pasteurized honey is purified through the heating process. Pasteurized honey reaches temperatures of at least 161°F. While this heating process kills off both bacteria and yeast cells alike, it also responsible for destroying much of the honey's valuable nutritional content. It also causes the honey to result in a darker color, although not all dark honey is the result of pasteurization (many times honey's color is determined by what type of flower source the honey is derived from).

- **Comb honey.** This is honey still packaged fresh inside the honeycomb. The honeycomb is collected, broken into pieces with the golden honey still inside, and packaged for distribution. The purchaser can then pour the honey from the comb, or eat the honey off the comb, chewing the comb as well.

- **Whipped or churned honey**. This is a soft, spreadable honey that has been formed out of the crystallization process. It is many times served on bagels or breakfast rolls, or whipped into desserts and frostings.

- **Dried honey**. In this truly solid form, excess moisture is pulled out of the honey to form a solid. Dried honey can be used as a garnish on gourmet desserts, or eaten whole as a sweet candy.

Grades of Honey

Much like the grading of eggs, honey is graded according to federal USDA guidelines. Honey grading is strictly voluntary, but is preferred and encouraged as it can offer much information about its quality.

Honey grades are based on four criteria:

- **Water content**. What is the percentage of water in the final honey product?

- **Flavor and aroma**. Should be consistent throughout and reflective of the source.

- **Absence of defects.** Should be absent of any overt defects, particles or artifacts.

- **Clarity.** Honey should be clear throughout, without anything that would affect its appearance. Color should be consistent, without "layering."

The best honeys are grade A, and honeys earning this grade will be marked as such on the bottle's label.

A brief description of grades and the guidelines they follows are:

- **Grade A.** This honey has a good flavor and aroma. It does not have caramelization or fermentation. It is clear of most artifacts, although sometimes trace pollen grains or spores can be found. Sometimes you will still notice tiny air bubbles in grade A honey. Water content is low (<18%).

- **Grade B.** This still has good flavor and aroma, although not as good as grade A. You may also notice slight caramelization and air bubbles. There may also be slightly more artifacts than grade A, but not enough to mark a noticeable difference. Water content is the same as grade A honey (<18%).

- **Grade C.** Grade C honey is reasonably good in flavor with an acceptable level of caramelization. Still not a noticeable amount of artifacts and air bubbles, but not enough to greatly impact its appearance. Slightly more water content than grades A or B honey, as you may notice it is not as thick.

- **Substandard Grade.** This grade fails the USDA guidelines for honey in any of the four categories. Substandard grade honey may be deemed too watery or contain obvious particles. It's flavor could be "off" or not clear enough for a higher rating.

What should I look for when purchasing ungraded honey?

When purchasing honey that does not indicate an USDA grade on the label, there are several indicators you can use for an indication of its quality.

For starters, honey should appear lightly golden (for most varieties) and remain consistent in its color. It should not have sediment at the bottom of the jar or look "layered" in its color throughout.

The best honey can be determined based on aroma, flavor and consistency. Honey should never have a rancid odor and, for the most part, should not contain noticeable particles floating within.

Occasionally, raw honey may contain an odd floater, such as a particle of comb or even a portion of bee wing. Since this honey has not gone through the pasteurization process and generally not been altered in any way, it has not had the opportunity for such specimens to be eliminated. However, this does not affect the goodness of the raw honey. In fact, raw honey has been known to offer the most in nutrient content.

An additional measure of honey's quality comes in its smoothness and pourability. You can insert a butter knife or frosting spatula directly into the bottle, coating it in honey. Remove the utensil and observe the honey draining back into the jar. Is it smooth and steady flowing? Or does it fall off in an uneven flow, or worse yet, fall off in clumps?

As you pour honey from the jar or bottle, the highest quality honey pours in a steady stream, instead of dripping out in clumps or formed droplets.

Storage and Shelf Life

Due to the sugar content in honey, it boasts an indefinite shelf life, and under normal circumstances does not go bad. Honey should be stored in an airtight jar or container out of the path of direct sunlight. Remember that honey, like chocolate, absorbs odors. It also absorbs moisture. Never store honey with anything that may alter its flavor and composition.

Honey does not need to be refrigerated, although it is okay to do so if the need arises. Refrigerated honey becomes thicker and may be a bit more cumbersome to use, but can easily be brought back to room temperature for simpler handling. Sometimes cold refrigerator temperatures cause crystallization to occur.

Over time, honey may become cloudy. This is the crystallization process taking place and will not change the flavor of the honey. If too much crystallization takes place and you wish to return it to its original liquid state, honey can be slowly heated and stirred to remove the crystallization. Just be cautious not to overhead the honey, as this will not only destroy much of its nutritional value, but also change its flavor.

And, if you ever have the need, yes honey can even be frozen without much effect to its vitamin and mineral content.

Honeys from Around the Globe

Because nectar from different flowers is different, honey is as different as the plants around the hive. The fragrances of the flowers which produce nectar flavors the honey which is made from it. Mostly, these are aromatic flower oils.

Generally, the lighter the honey, the lighter and more delicate its flavor. The darker the honey, the more intense the flavor. For example, sweet clover honey is light golden in color and flavor, while buckwheat honey is dark in color and heavy in flavor.

Honey's color varies from clear, almost water-white, to nearly black.

Most tropical honey is thin; most northern honey is thick.

The clover honey of Ohio, Michigan and New York is the standard for most of the industry. It possesses the golden color, taste and consistency most people associate with first class honey.

Other geographical areas are known for the special honeys they produce, as well. Some of the best known honeys are:

Texas produces two especially fragrant honeys, mesquite and grapefruit blossom. The grapefruit honey has a wonderful, spicy fragrance and flavor.

New England's raspberry honey is especially fragrant; its locust honey is more subtle in flavor.

Washington and Oregon produce light, subtly flavored, fireweed honey.

West Virginia, Ohio and Michigan are known for their dark, strongly flavored, buckwheat honey. It is dark, intense, rich and thick, with a flavor somewhat like that of malt.

Alabama is the home of a pale, delicate honey from cotton blossom nectar.

California markets more honey than any other state. Some of its best honeys are from the nectars of mountain sage, alfalfa, orange blossoms, mountain lilac, lima bean blossoms and the star thistle.

Pale, straw-colored orange blossom honey is produced in many citrus growing areas. It carries the distinctive aroma of blooming citrus and is an especially syrupy honey. Some people find it too sweet-tasting.

Florida's tupelo honey is one of the most aromatic of all the honeys. Florida also is produces mangrove and palm honey.

Basswood honey is produced by some northwestern states. This peppermint-tasting honey has a flavor that is very penetrating. It taints other honeys, even when blended with other strong flavors.

And honey's individuality continues across the globe:

Some honeys from the West Indies are based on the nectar of tropical swamp flowers. It is quite dark in color and apt to be bitter. Other West Indian honey is made from tobacco blossom nectar and has the rich flavor of these plants.

Grasse, France enjoys world renown for its jasmine flavored honey. Other French regions are known for a delicate rosemary flavored honey and a lovely sea-green honey made from gooseberry bush or sycamore tree nectar. This country is also famous for its lavender honey.

Spain is known for its pale amber-colored rosemary honey. Considered too fine a honey for most cooking, it is usually served as a spread for bread. This superb honey is sometimes used as the base for turron, a fondant type of candy popular in Spain and other Mediterranean and North African countries.

Scotland is best known for its heather honey. It is very thick and aromatic, with a purplish cast to it. Heather honey is considered very healthful because of its higher than average mineral content.

Heather honey can also be reddish brown, deep amber or even ruby-red. Darker colored varieties are apt to be a bit bitter.

Cuba produces a mixed wildflower honey that has a distinctive, medium-strong aroma and taste.

Australia's eucalyptus honey is exceptionally good for external healing and for boosting general health. This golden brown honey can be somewhat bitter. Honey from the blossoms of the white gum tree is milder.

Guatemala's coffee plantations market a coffee flavored honey.

India produces a delicate, lightly aromatic honey made from lotus blossom nectar.

Some call acacia the most magnificent of all the kinds of honey. The very best is produced in Hungary. This pale, almost clear honey carries the aromatic perfume of acacia flowers.

Acacia honey is one of the sweetest, and one of the most expensive honeys.

Italy markets a dark brown, mildly astringent chestnut honey and one from the black locust.

Greece produces an elegant rose honey, but is much better known for its thyme honey. Throughout the ages, poets have written of the divine nature of honey made from the wild thyme growing on the mountains east of Athens. Sicily is also famous for its rich, golden thyme honey.

Non "Nectar" Honey?
Honey comes in as many flavors as there are flowers and nectar -- and in a few not seen in nature! Chocolate

flavored honey has been found in hives near a chocolate candy factory. And, Coca-Cola® flavored honey was made by bees feeding on the liquid left in discarded soda cans.

There's even pine-flavored honey! Most well-known in Germany, bees make it from honeydew they find on pine trees. Even though the pine does not produce a nectar-bearing flower, bees still make honey from a nectar that can sometimes be found on pine trees.

When insects (such as aphids) feed on pine sap, they excrete honeydew onto the pine needles. This honeydew is then gathered by bees for honey. Pine honey is very dark and intensely flavored, with a medicinal sort of taste.

Best Honey Producing Plants

Some flowering plants produce more nectar than others, making it easier for bees to gather. Hyssop is a good plant to have around for honey, because it makes a lot of nectar for the bees.

Some other plants that produce good honey are:

- Alfalfa
- Apple
- Aster
- Basil
- Bergamont
- Blackberry
- Borage
- Butterfly weed

- Catnip
- Chamomile
- Cherry
- Chicory
- Crocus
- Currant
- Dandelion
- Gooseberry
- Fennel
- Goldenrod
- Ground ivy
- Lime
- Lemon balm
- Marigold
- Milkweed
- Mint
- Palmetto
- Persimmon
- Quince
- Sunflower
- Tulip tree
- Willow

Poisonous Honey

Honey produced from certain types of plants is considered poisonous. Specific toxins, called grayanotoxins, can be found in plants such as rhododendrons and azaleas. The honey that is made from these plants' nectar produces this toxic chemical and can bring about a very rare, but dangerous poisonous reaction called grayanotoxin poisoning (sometimes referred to as honey intoxication).

Grayanotoxin poisoning can cause heavy perspiration, vomiting, dizziness, loss of coordination, severe muscle weakness and a dropping of blood pressure. Very rarely is grayanotoxin poisoning life threatening and usually symptoms end within a day.

One of the earliest reports of poisonous honey came from a general in the army of the ancient Greeks. Xenophon was leading about 10,000 soldiers in a retreat from fighting in Persia. They camped in the Pontus area of Turkey. Within a few hours of encampment his soldiers were suffering so much from vomiting and diarrhea they could not stand up.

Xenophon's soldiers recovered in about three days and resumed their retreat. Their sickness was blamed on the local honey, made from the nectar of a certain rhododendron plant. Greek historians also wrote about other encounters with poisonous honey from rhododendrons and azalea plants.

Additional reports of toxic honey have come from Old Persia, Corsica, Russia, Japan, Turkey and even Philadelphia, Pennsylvania right here in the United States.

For the most part, toxic honey comes from some varieties of rhododendron and azalea plants. But not all plants, even though considered poisonous, produce poisonous honey. For example, honey derived from bees obtaining nectar from the poison ivy plant is not poisonous, and can be eaten without concern.

When obtaining honey from a questionable source, great care should be taken to avoid honey produced from plant varieties such as rhododendrons, azaleas and oleanders. The honey produced from these plants is considered toxic and should not be eaten.

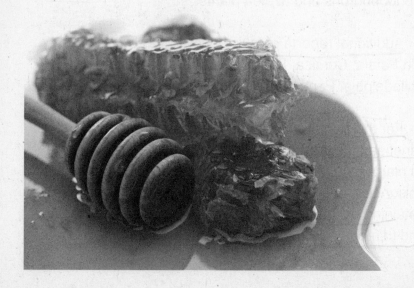

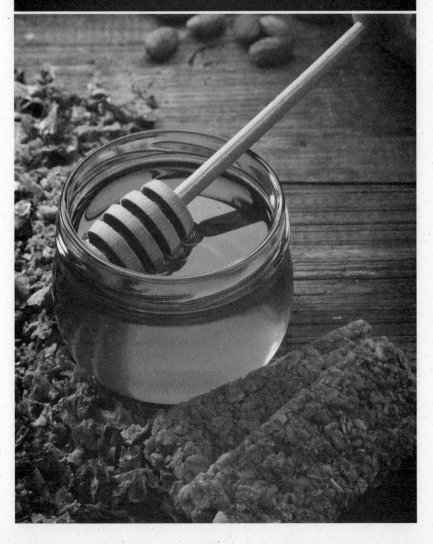

CHAPTER THREE

Bees & Honey Production: How it All Works

Mankind's continuing fascination with the bee is part fear and part love. Fear of the bee's sting and love of honey's wonderful sweetness have guided man's relationship with bees for ages.

Bees have played a substantial role in the development of man. European immigrants brought the honeybee to North America. Wherever they went, bees went too. America's Indians soon came to consider honeybees a sign of the coming of the white man.

Now, North America is seeing the advance of another bee, the African honey bee. This "bee with an attitude problem" has reached the lower Rio Grande Valley in Texas. They are interbreeding with local bees, and slowly advancing across the country. This bee is more aggressive, more protective of its nest, than the more peaceful honeybee.

The Honey Makers
Honeybees are social insects. 50,000 (or more) often live and work together in a unique display of community cooperation. Each insect has a specific duty in maintaining the hive.

A hive is made up of a single queen and many drones and workers. For each queen there are 100s of drones and 1,000s of workers.

The queen is an egg laying machine. She lays up to 2,000 eggs a day, over a 3 to 5 year life span. The hive's worker bees take care of nurturing eggs into full grown bees.

Workers seal the queen's eggs in amazing six-sided wax cells. A single egg is placed in each cell. Larva, a little white worm, hatches out of each egg in about 3 days. It is fed until it grows enough to completely fill its little wax cell. Then, workers seal the worm in by capping the cell with wax.

Then a magical metamorphosis takes place. The helpless little wormlike creature develops wings and legs – it becomes a honeybee.

Eggs which have been fertilized produce female bees (workers) and unfertilized eggs produce male bees (drones). If a developing female bee is well-fed with "royal jelly," a queen bee is produced.

Drones are pretty much helpless, and depend on other bees for food. Their only purpose is to fertilize a new queen, should something happen to the current one. Drones are only fed during summer when it is easy for the hive to support them.

Worker bees are sterile females. (They were not fed royal jelly in the larva stage.) Workers have wax glands on the bottom of their abdomens and pollen baskets on their hind legs. They produce the honey and beeswax for the hive.

Worker bees live for 4 to 5 weeks in the summer and longer in the winter, when the hive is mostly quiet. Each has a specific job to do, one that changes with age, sort of a bee version of the "seniority system." Each worker bee starts out in housekeeping and eventually becomes a forager.

Each worker honeybee has a specific job cycle they are responsible for to help maintain a healthy hive:

- **Housekeeper**. As soon as the larva completes its metamorphosis and chews its way out of the wax cell, it begins its housekeeping duties by cleaning out empty cells for reuse.

- **Nurse**. From the third day of life to about the tenth, nurse workers feed larva honey and small amounts of royal jelly, a special food that can turn a sterile female into a new queen.

- **Builder** - Builder bees are responsible for building new wax cells and repairing used or damaged ones.

- **Honey maker**. These bees store nectar and pollen brought in by other bees and turn nectar into finished honey.

- **Guard**. Guard bees use antennae (like airport metal detectors) to examine bees returning to the hive. Guard bees can distinguish whether or not an approaching bee belongs to their particular hive. (Only drones can go to neighboring hives, for crossbreeding, to keep the species diversified).

- **Forager**. The most mature, skilled bees are foragers. These bees are responsible for gathering pollen and nectar for the hive.

Queens are usually produced in late spring. The old queen takes some of the workers and flies off to a new location. The bees who follow her produce a "swarm."

When the queen is gone, new queens are produced. The first queen out of her cell kills all the other developing queens. She then flies out of the hive and the drones follow her. The queen mates with several drones over a period of a few days. Her entire lifetime production of eggs is fertilized during this period.

The queen's only duty is to lay eggs. Each egg is about 1/16 of an inch in length, and she lays one every few seconds, all around the clock.

Nurse bees secrete a nutrient-filled food called "royal jelly." Mostly, it is for feeding the queen bee. Workers and drones eat pollen and honey.

Occasionally a small creature, such as a caterpillar or mouse, will invade a hive. The bees sting it to death but are not strong enough to drag the corpse back out of the hive. To keep these dead intruders from rotting and contaminating the entire hive, the bees seal them in a resin they find in the bark of trees and leave the body where it lies.

Beekeeping

Bees do not have strong jaws, so they are not able to hollow out places, such as trees or logs, for their hives. Instead, they build wax chambers in natural cavities.

Bees need an area that is protected from rain, wind and snow. They tend to nest in hollow tree trunks, rock clefts, and occasionally, the hollow walls of buildings.

More efficient shelters are provided by beekeepers. Artificial hives make it easier for bees to produce honey and easier for the beekeeper to remove it.

Bees are able to make more honey than they need to get through the winter. So, beekeepers are able to safely remove much of what they produce.

First, the beekeeper stuns the bees with smoke. When the first smoke enters the hive, the bees rush to honey cells and gorge themselves. These full bees are less alert and are less likely to sting. The keeper puts more smoke into the hive, then opens it and removes part of the honey.

Pollen

Pollen is necessary for raising the bees' larvae. It contains protein, B vitamins, riboflavin, pantothenic acid and much more.

Pollen comes in a rainbow of colors. It varies from plant to plant. Bees tend to concentrate on one kind of flower at time, so pollen stored in different parts of the hive will be colored differently.

Some plants and their pollen colors follow:

- Dandelion is orange
- Apple is yellow or green
- White clover is pale brown
- Fireweed is light blue
- Poppy is black

Bees seem to be most attracted to the pollen and nectar of blue flowers. Their favorite sources of pollen and nectar are fruit trees, clover, dandelions, lavender, daisies and dahlias.

Bee Legend and Lore

As you can see, the world of bees is both complicated and fascinating in nature. It is with this fascination that fact has developed into amazing folk lore and legend throughout the ages. It seems every civilization has offered its own contribution to the library of bee legend and lore.

Because Hindus consider honey the food of the gods, they hold a piece of a plant they considered to be sacred in their hands when taking honey out of hives. This is supposed to protect them from being stung. The plant, called toolsy (or holy basil), is very aromatic.

In some parts of the world it is believed rubbing hot water and wine on hives will keep bees from swarming.

Mites and other parasites of bees can be killed by fumigating the hive with burnt asses' dung.

Did you know the native bee of Australia is stingless?

There were several Old Irish laws that included fines for wantonly killing bees.

European beekeepers say one should give some honey to their neighbors. This is because the bees probably used some of the neighbors' nectar in making the honey in the first place. Sharing this year is supposed to ensure a good harvest next year.

Some say they can call swarming bees with a simple whistle. Others claim they can attract them by beating on pans or metal objects, or by ringing bells.

Bees can be bothered by mites. These tiny parasites suck nutrients from bees, leaving them weak and frail, and virtually defenseless.

Honey bears destroy hives, wasps and ants. Beetles eat honey, and caterpillars eat beeswax. And so bees have stingers to protect their hives. They tend to sting when alerted by strange odors, such as human perspiration, tobacco smoke, alcohol, onions, garlic, bright colors and perfume.

Although some bees are instinctively more aggressive than others, usually a bee only stings to defend itself or its home. When near a hive, avoid stings by wearing neutral colors and moving slowly and quietly. If you are stung by a bee, the leaves of mallow, mint, lemon balm or ivy can be rubbed on the skin to soothe the hurt. Scratching the sting should be avoided, as this will prolong any itchy reaction.

Scottish tradition says it is unlucky to buy bees. It is better to barter for them.

Welsh folklore promises that no one will have good luck with purchased bees. A hive should be given for good luck to come to the household.

In Ireland it is said bees should only be bought with money that was honestly earned by hard work.

Folks in the northern countries of England say that if a bee swarm lands on dead wood, someone in the family of the owner of the bees will die.

Bees are encouraged to make lots of honey by sprinkling their hives with fresh milk and children's urine.

If you put the liver of a white falcon in a beehive, the bees with flourish.

To ensure that a colony of bees does well, put a bear's eye in their hive.

If you do not give honey to a sick person who requests it, your bees will stop making honey.

Just for Fun

If a swarm of bees settles on your home, you will have good fortune. If they make a nest in the eaves, it is even better luck.

Many old-timers in England and Scotland believe bees hum at midnight on Christmas Eve.

The original Old English version of the phrase, "A bee in your bonnet" projects an entirely different meaning — "There's a maggot in your head."

If the owner of a hive of bees is miserly, the bees will not work hard. Bees will not prosper if owned by a quarrelsome family. And, stolen bees will surely die.

Folklore dictates that if there is a death in the family, the family's bees must be told about it. Be sure and knock on the bees' hive 3 times before telling them about the death. Then ask them to please stay and work for the new master.

When a swarm of bees lands on a tree branch, that piece of wood will have magic qualities.

Bees will surely sting you if you do not talk politely to them.

Never count your bee hive, it will bring bad luck. If you put some empty hives among the working ones, it will confuse anyone trying to count them.

Never swear at bees. They will either sicken and die or sting you. If you quarrel over bees, they will be so sad they will die.

Because bees are in touch with the next world, when one stings you, it means you have a relative in Purgatory who has sent the bee to remind you to pray for them.

If a queen bee lands on you, death will come very soon. But if you dream about bees, you can expect to make a good profit, very soon.

When a servant dreams of a bee swarm, it means that person will soon be without a job.

If a whole lot of noisy bees appear in your dream, someone is gossiping about you.

It is said that when the devil saw God create bees, he tried to make some, too. The bees created by the devil became wasps.

Honeybees cannot feed on the sweet nectar of the red clover plant because it is located too deep in the blossom. It is said this is the bees' punishment for not keeping the Sabbath.

To take honey without being stung, do not speak on the day you open the hive.

The African honey-bird will lead you to the hollow tree where honey can be found, but you must leave some of the honey for the bird. Otherwise, the next time the bird will lead you to where a snake is waiting.

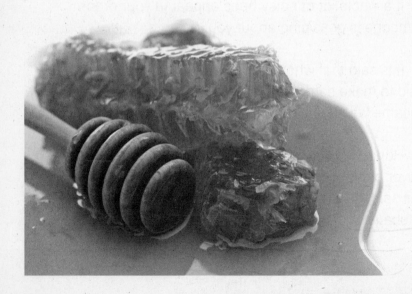

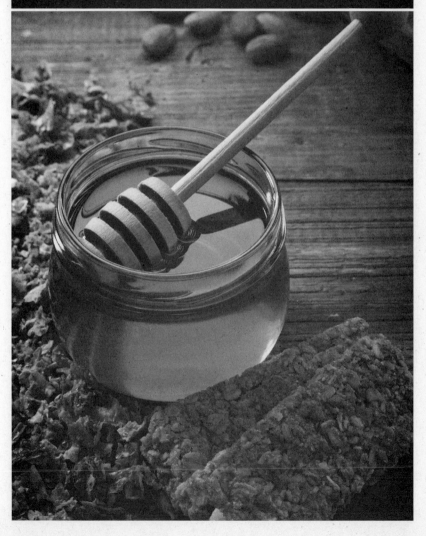

CHAPTER FOUR

Science Behind the Sweetness

Consider a few recent news excerpts about honey's medicinal prospects:

> *England's prestigious Journal of the Royal Society of Medicine carries a letter calling honey "a remedy rediscovered..."*

> *A dental surgeon reports on using honey as an after-surgery dressing for an impacted molar...*

> *Honey outperforms conventional dressings in healing burns...*

Honey is being used in hospitals and tested in science laboratories all across the world. One of the things researchers are proving is that honey does contain healing properties.

Researchers are beginning to understand more about how and why honey seems to have so much to offer in healing, even though most of the scientific analysis which has been done on honey leaves nearly 3% of it labeled as "unclassified."

Honey is an active fighter against both bacteria and fungus, it fights both staphylococcus and streptococcus, all the while not harming healthy tissue.

Throughout time, and in nations across the world, honey has been a staple in folk medicine. There have been many health claims made for it. It has been said to be a remedy for a slew of common ailments and discomforts.

A few of those ailments include:

- Arthritis
- Bronchitis
- Cancer
- Diabetes
- Goiter
- Insomnia
- Neuritis
- Burns
- Cuts
- Scrapes
- Wounds
- Surgical incisions

It is also said to lift the spirit and energize the body.

Many scientific studies are under way, all attempting to either prove or disprove the idea that faith in honey as a healing agent is merited. Early results show honey inhibits the growth of many kinds of harmful microbes. And, it is active against kinds that are resistant to the more usual drug-based antimicrobial agents.

The American Journal of Surgery reported that a study indicated wounds treated with regular, commercial honey healed faster than those without it.

The Journal put it this way, "...honey seems to accelerate wound healing...due to its energy-producing properties...our results suggest that honey....accelerates the healing process."

In one test conducted by a university hospital, 98% of ulcerated lesions showed "remarkable improvement" after being spread with honey.

A British surgeon reports he used honey to treat a deep surgical incision. He packed the cavity each day with granulated honey and topped it with dry gauze. He found that not only did the incision heal quickly, the honey did not irritate the surrounding skin tissue as many other treatments and solutions might have.

The surgeon's conclusion was that honey is sterile, attacks bacteria, is nutritive, cheap, easy to obtain and extremely effective.

Another reason hospitals find honey to be a superb surgical dressing is that is does not stick to skin or wound surfaces. Honey is an instant "fit" for irregular surfaces or jagged edges. And, when honey touches healthy skin there is no danger of irritation (as happens with some of the more traditional medicinal products).

Honey is currently being used with great success on:

- Amputations
- Varicose ulcers
- Chronic osteomyelitis (bone infections)
- Dental infections and abscesses
- Gangrenous patients
- Hospital and nursing home patients with painful bedsores
- Post-operative incision healing

- Burn and scald victims
- Skin graft preservation
- Soak for cornea transplants
- Surgical dressing
- Anti-fungal cream
- Anti-inflammatory illnesses
- Reduce the risk of heart disease
- Improving the effectiveness of some cancer fighting medications
- Anti-proliferate agent
- Arthritic symptoms

One university teaching hospital tested honey, in a controlled study, as a treatment for gangrene. Some patients were treated with topical applications of honey, others were treated with a more conventional approach.

The results were exciting. Patients treated with honey felt better sooner. No one treated with honey died (3 patients who did not receive honey did die), treatment was much less expensive and surgical procedures were avoided, so patients were not required to undergo anesthesia.

Researchers expect their results to revolutionize the way some gangrene is treated.

And more studies are being conducted all over the world.

According to research at Cairo University, dental abscesses and bone infections have been successfully treated by packing them with honey.

The Australian & New Zealand Journal of Obstetrics & Gynecology reports honey is useful as an alternative way to manage abdominal wounds. In this study, they successfully tested honey on infected Caesarean section patients.

Incisions were smeared with honey and covered with tape – instead of the normal practice of being redressed and resutured. In all cases, honey promoted complete healing within two weeks. Physicians were pleased, as honey treatment is inexpensive and avoids the need to resuture wounds, which requires the administration of general anesthesia.

Honey, according to another university study, is effective as an ulcer dressing. It gives good control of infection because of its ability to attract moisture. And, its natural hydrogen peroxide inhibits bacteria growth.

Honey also fights infection with substances the university researchers were unable to positively identify. These unrecognizable ingredients were thought to be from the flowers which provided nectar for the honey's production.

Antibacterial action of honey varies, depending upon the kind of nectar that is was produced from. Manuka honey, in a recent test, completely inhibited the growth of staph – and 6 other types of major wound infecting bacteria.

Researchers say, "Honey is thus an ideal topical wound dressing agent in surgical infections, burns and wound infections."

They felt unprocessed raw honey did the best job of treating infection. It inhibited most fungi and bacteria.

Unpasteurized honey's antibacterial activity was greatest when it was from a single type of flower, rather than a mix of nectars. Honey made from mixed flower nectar was much less effective.

High antibacterial activity was found in honey made from the blossoms of manuka, heather and some members of the borage family.

Corneas to be used for transplanting are very delicate and difficult to preserve. Surgeons have found they can be saved or their usefulness prolonged during transportation by storing them in a honey solution.

Skin grafts, too, have been preserved by soaking them in a solution containing honey, allowing them to stay supple and useful longer.

Honey has even been shown to promote the healing of ulcers in leprosy patients.

Tests have shown that some cancer incisions heal better if given a coating of honey.

Researchers at the American Health Foundation recently announced that a substance found in honeybee hives inhibits the development of precancerous colon changes. It is hoped that research findings such as these will soon be turned into useful remedies, and the research is ongoing.

Pressure or bed sores, one of the worst threats to the elderly, have been shown to heal after being covered in honey. Honey causes less pain and encourages faster healing than many drug-based salves. It also helps to get rid of the odor associated with many long-established bed sores.

Honey has been shown to be antibacterial, so it is an effective agent against salmonella, the bacteria often found in poultry.

Honey is effective in keeping the growth of E. coli in check, a troublesome bacteria being found more and more in commercially-prepared foods. It is also effective against several types of fungus.

According to Science News, honey is:

- Antifungal
- Antibacterial
- Anti-inflammatory
- Antiproliferative
- Able to make cancer-fighting drugs more effective

Several broad spectrum antibiotics, called tetracyclines, have been found to occur naturally in honey. A few of these include:

- Chlorotetracycline
- Demeclocycline
- Demethylchlortetracycline
- Doxycycline
- Methacycline
- Minocycline
- Oxytetracycline

Nutrition

Honey, by nature, is rich in carbohydrates. It contains several different types of carbohydrates used by the body for quick energy. It has monosaccharides, disaccharides and trisaccharides.

Monosaccharides are the most basic and most simple form of sugar. Disaccharides are the sugar molecules made up of the combination of two monosaccharides, while trisaccharides are the molecules made up of three monosaccharides. Why is this important as far as diet is concerned? Because each plays an important role in dietary function in our human body. And honey is found to contain each of these!

After consuming honey, it is rapidly absorbed into the bloodstream. Many believe it is less likely than refined sugar to cause a repeated craving for sugar. Early tests also confirm this belief.

There is also some protein found in honey. A total of 19 different proteins were found in a single variety of Australian honey. Most of the protein is in pollen grains found floating within the honey itself.

Honey is also not only a fat free food, but also cholesterol free.

It is a natural sweetener, free from over processing and chemical additives found in so many of today's off-the-grocery-shelf sweetening agents. It is great for enhancing the body's immune system and is also contains antioxidant properties. Antioxidants are important in fighting free-radicals in the body which cause cancer.

Honey also contains many important vitamins and minerals the human body needs on a daily basis.

Honey vs. Sugar

So, the question has long been asked, "Which is better, honey or sugar?"

Much research has been done into the question of whether honey or sugar is the better, more nutritious choice of sweetener. After many studies, the verdict is clear that honey is a superb choice as an all natural sweetener.

When used in comparison with white, refined table sugar, honey boasts numerous health benefits sugar does not.

In addition to its natural healing properties, honey does contain antioxidants that help the body fight many types of cancers, while antioxidants are not present in white sugar. Neither does table sugar contain the vitamins, mineral and enzymes present in natural honey.

Table sugar is considered a highly processed and a highly refined food. And some researchers consider sugar void of any real nutritional benefit whatsoever.

Sugar has been shown to raise blood sugar levels at a higher rate than honey when identical amounts are used. In fact, some scientific studies have shown that honey, unlike table sugar, can actually improve the body's function in processing glucose and aid the body in digestion.

And, because honey is a concentrated sweetener, much sweeter than regular refined table sugar, less honey is required to achieve the same level of sweetness. Honey is also easier for the body to digest than sugar. So, while honey possesses countless natural healing properties, one can also reap the benefits of the healthy, natural goodness of eating honey over table sugar as well.

A word of caution. While honey is naturally both fat-free and cholesterol-free, care should be taken not to eat too much of a good thing where weight loss and overall caloric intake is concerned. While honey makes a fantastic substitution for sugar and other sweeteners, it is still relatively high in calories. Honey contains about 64 calories in a tablespoon, while highly processed table sugar boasts about 46. But remember you will need less honey than white sugar to sweeten the same drink or confection So, just don't mistake fat-free with calorie-free.

What about Honey and Diabetes?

So what about honey as it relates to diabetic patients and their unique needs? Is honey a safe alternative to sugar for those people?

Surprisingly, new research is indicating that honey might actually be a healthier alternative to table sugar for people suffering from diabetes. As discussed earlier, while honey does contain slightly more calories than refined table sugar, the biggest difference is in the way your body handles the two sweeteners.

When sugary substances are consumed, it rapidly finds its way into the bloodstream, causing an immediate rise or "spike" in glucose levels. But, because honey consists of two simple sugars, glucose and fructose, it is absorbed into the system at a much slower rate. Honey has been found to raise blood sugar levels slower, over a more drawn out period of time.

Because honey takes a more prolonged, gradual approach to raising glucose levels in the bloodstream, the body may not require the addition of mass quantities of insulin. This can be extremely beneficial, as it tends to avoid the rapid spike in blood glucose levels associated with type 2 diabetes.

One indicator of this fact lies in honey's glycemic rating. Honey scores a moderate 55 in comparison to table sugar's rating of a high 100. (The glycemic scale runs from 0-100, with foods scoring 100 having the most rapid rise in blood sugar levels).

But, every body is different and every body processes foods differently. Continue to check blood glucose levels to ensure safety.

This more moderate and prolonged absorption into the system may make honey a better sweetening option for diabetics.

As always, proper care should be taken when incorporating honey into the diabetic diet. Honey still must be considered for its carbohydrate amounts as well as its glycemic implications. But this may offer diabetes sufferers a springboard for discussion with health care providers into the beneficial aspects of the honey option in relation to their disease.

Hypoglycemia

In addition to being an alternative for diabetics, honey can also be used to stabilize blood sugar levels in those suffering from hypoglycemia. Just a single tablespoonful of honey can be used to safely raise low blood sugar levels back to within a safe range for hypoglycemic.

Burns

Because of honey's natural antibacterial and antimicrobial properties, it can be a very useful treatment when applied topically to burns and scalds. Not only can honey fight the onset of bacterial infections of damaged burn tissue, but studies have found it also promotes more rapid healing of skin tissue while leaving behind less scarring.

Honey is easy to put on wounds and burns, especially with wet fingers. It flows easily into awkward places and covers irregular wound edges. As honey is diluted by moisture from the injury, it naturally produces hydrogen peroxide, which attacks bacteria.

Honey heals burns with less scarring because there is less likelihood of infection, and because honey's hygroscopic action keeps burns from drying out.

The British Journal of Surgery reports these findings from a controlled study of honey as a dressing for burns:

- 91% of honey-treated burns became sterile within 7 days

- 7% of burns receiving standard treatment were sterile within 7 days

- 87% of honey-treated wounds healed within 15 days

- 10% of burns receiving standard treatment healed within 15 days

- Patients with honey-treated burns reported less pain

- Patients with honey-treated burns had less scarring and deformity

In addition to its lower cost and easy availability, these researchers called honey "…an ideal dressing in the treatment of burns."

Studies continue into how honey can be safely used in the treatment of burn patients. Expect great strides in this area of treatment in the future.

Digestion

Honey is used as a remedy for indigestion because it is soothing to the membranes of the digestive tract. It is easily and quickly absorbed, so it delivers the body a maximum amount of energy for a minimum amount of digestive work.

Honey is a traditional treatment for indigestion. It has now been demonstrated by researchers that a major cause of indigestion, helicobacter pylori, has its growth stopped by dilute solutions of honey.

Honey is also a natural, gentle laxative.

Some medical authorities recommend honey as a food for heart patients and for those who have had strokes and major surgeries. Its unique combination of sugars is easy for exhausted bodies to use, and the extra nitrogen it proves to the body is healing.

The invertase in honey, especially, has been recommended for those who are sick or frail.

Honey also contains acetylcholine. This chemical can stimulate the heart, increase metabolism rates and improve blood circulation.

Tests show that acetylcholine, a chemical found in honey, stimulates the digestive organs and kidneys, as well.

Honey and Alcohol Consumption

Home remedies for hangovers have traditionally included honey. Now researchers are finding out why. Fructose, a sugar in honey, speeds up oxidation of alcohol by the body's liver.

Actually, honey is more effective as a hangover remedy than pure fructose. It is thought this is because honey contains enzymes which also help with oxidation of alcohol.

Some investigators think taking honey before drinking alcohol may act as a hangover preventative. (It is especially effective when taken with a source of vitamin C, such as lemon juice.)

Honey has been used to protect the stomach from the damage of alcohol. A test showed that having honey in the stomach 30 minutes before alcohol reached it produced an 80% protection rate (for gastric lesions). This suggests honey can be useful in reducing, or even preventing, stomach damage caused by alcohol.

Allergies

Honey has long been touted as a remedy for those suffering from allergies. While tests are still ongoing, many believe honey eaten from local sources can be beneficial to combating seasonal allergies.

As we've discussed in previous chapters, honey is not a pristine food, but contains many "artifacts". One of those artifacts found in honey is pollen spores. The theory is that when honey is taken from localities in the same surrounding area as allergy sufferers, the honey contains the very same type of pollen spores the allergy sufferer is allergic to. (By local honey, we are referring to honey derived from beehives within a few miles of the sufferer.) Because eating local honey exposes the sufferer to pollen spores in very tiny amounts, the body has an opportunity to build its immune systems and develop a response to the allergen. Very much like the way a child gets a vaccine as a preventative measure against certain diseases. The child receives a small dose of the disease, so that the body can build a defense against it. This process of exposure is called immunotherapy.

In order to receive the most benefit from local honey, one should make an effort to obtain local honey that is still in its raw, or most natural, fresh-from-the-hive, state.

While the verdict is still out on the effectiveness of this exposure, more and more people are eating honey from local hives as a preventative measure for many types of seasonal allergies.

New tests show hay fever symptoms really can be eased by chewing fresh beeswax.

The British Journal of Clinical Pharmacology tells of experiments which tested homeopathic honey remedies for allergies. More than 65% of those tested found relief by taking drops of very highly diluted honey.

It has now been revealed that people who have had allergic reactions after eating honey were more likely reacting to the pollen in the honey. These people are usually able to switch to consuming a honey derived from other kinds of plants.

Of all the honey-allergy sufferers in recent tests, 3/4 were allergic to dandelion honey, and more than half had a reaction to multiple flower honeys.

Even more...
Honey is an important ingredient in many commercial cough mixes. Treat a ticklish throat with honey and lemon juice, honey and apple cider vinegar, honey and garlic and nutmeg.

When weather or water causes chapped hands or lips, it appears honey is better at healing them than oily creams.

Children and Honey
One of the best reasons to use honey on children's injuries is that it is nontoxic. If little ones get it in their mouths, there is no worry about the child ingesting harmful chemical salves or lotions.

A few pats of honey on children's chapped or irritated skin can hasten healing. It is gentle enough for their delicate skin.

The British Medical Journal says honey is helpful in preventing dehydration in children. It has also been shown to shorten the duration of bacterial diarrhea.

Warning! Never give honey to a child who is less than 1 year old! This is due to the possibility of infant botulism and should always be avoided.

The New Athletic Enhancer

Serious sport enthusiasts have long touted the significance of loading up on high carbohydrate-type foods prior to a sporting event. It is not uncommon for athletes to load up on simple carbohydrates in an attempt to give themselves a quick energy boost prior to games or competitions. The problem with many quick boost carbohydrates is that the easily digested food enters the body too rapidly, and athletes can find themselves quickly coming off a sugar "high" and actually plummeting energy-wise in the process.

When the body absorbs simple sugars too quickly, the pancreas releases insulin to help properly regulate the body's blood sugar level. This quick release of insulin can sometimes leave athletes with the opposite effect, feeling their energy levels depleted after the initial burst of energy. Most simple carbohydrates, like sugar, are just absorbed into the blood stream too quickly to be of any long term help.

Now researchers are looking at honey as a the new energy boost for athletes. While honey is still very high in energy-producing carbohydrates, it is slower than sugar to be digested, thus entering the blood stream at a much slower rate. This gives the athlete a prolonged surge in energy, rather than an initial boost that quickly fades leaving the athlete sapped of energy. Researchers even refer to this prolonged boost as something of a 'time-released' fuel for the body's muscles.

This works because honey is made up of two sugars, sucrose and fructose, that take longer to digest than just plain sugar, which some sports enhancing drinks and gels are comprised of. The slower release into the body means the pancreas does not need to release large, concentrated amounts of insulin at one time.

And, different from the quick-boost effect of other foods, honey has been shown to keep the body's energy levels up for a greater length of time. Some studies indicate this boost in energy to last for nearly two hours post consumption.

One specific study indicated that long distance cyclists who were given honey in the place of either a competing energy booster or a placebo showed a significant increase in power and endurance than their competitors.

In addition, honey has also been shown to be effective in aiding post-workout recovery to help replenish and rebuild muscles after tough workouts.

So, how much honey does one need to receive this energy boost? Researchers believe about 2 tablespoons will do the trick. It can be eaten by itself, or mixed into a water beverage for a drink on the go.

Honey Can be Dangerous

It has been said "You are what you eat." Well, honey is what a bee eats! And sometimes bees feed on rhododendron nectar. Some rhododendron nectar has been found to cause illness, because it contains grayanotoxins.

Grayanotoxins are toxins found in the Ericaceae plant family. This can include rhododendrons and azaleas, among others. As bees feed on the nectar found in these plants, the poisonous toxins are then transmitted into the honey those bees produce.

This is the same honey that caused ancient Greek soldiers to get sick during their march through Turkey. The plant which produces this "mad" nectar is called "rhododendron ponticum." It can be found throughout areas in Turkey, Japan, Brazil, Europe and even in some parts of North America.

Two tablespoons of honey with grayanotoxins can cause illness.

The Journal of the American Medical Association reports there were 16 cases of "mad honey" poisoning in a two-year period. It is not usually fatal, but can cause temporary breathing problems or a sudden drop in blood pressure.

Some honey has been found to carry Clostridium botulinum spores. These are especially dangerous to infants, and is why babies should not be given honey.

All honey does not contain botulinum spores. But, because of the danger posed by botulism poisoning, infants under 1 year of age SHOULD NEVER BE GIVEN HONEY.

When pesticides are used on pasture lands where bees forage, they can get into the honey. One report tells of cyanide containing pesticides being used to kill bees. The poison showed up in honey made by other bees in that area.

Commercial honey is tested for insecticide residues, to keep it safe. Usually, more of these chemicals are stored in the beeswax than in the honey itself.

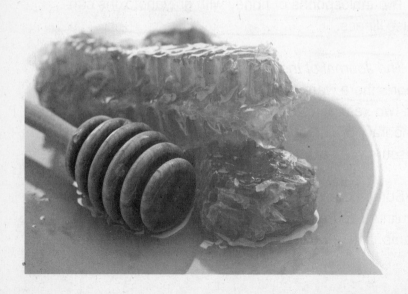

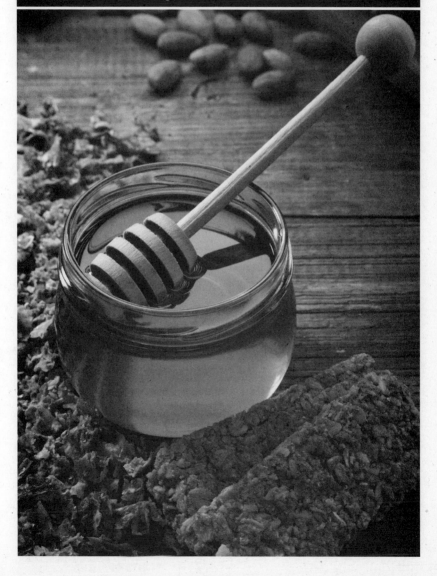

CHAPTER FIVE
More from the Hive

Honey is sweet, fast energy. It contains sugars that can enter the bloodstream in as little as 10 minutes. According to the Department of Agriculture's nutritionist, the sweet "enhances intestinal absorption of calcium." Calcium supplements taken at the same time as honey are absorbed 25% better than those taken without it.

And bees offer even more! Other products from the beehive include pollen, royal jelly, propolis and beeswax. These by-products of honey production are much more expensive than honey. They are also much more concentrated.

Pollen Power

Bee pollen is the delicate dust bees collect on their legs while foraging for sweet nectar. It has been credited with being able to promote healing and long life because it is such a nutrient packed food.

Sometimes, pollen is called "bee bread." Most pollen grains look like golden dust and are loaded with proteins. They are gathered by bees that return to the hive looking as if they are wearing wide yellow pantaloons.

Pollen contains vitamins, minerals, amino acids, proteins and trace elements. When the bees finish with pollen, it is covered with a barrier that helps preserve it.

Grains of pollen can be added to the diet as an aid in treating hay fever, as can chewed honeycomb. They act as immunizing agents. To be effective, the pollen must come from hives in the area where the person being treated lives. That way, the pollen is from the plants that cause the person's hay fever.

One way pollen is used for hay fever is to take some of it every day during the month just before hay fever season.

Eat pollen by sprinkling it on cereal, stirring it into juices, or adding it to salad dressings. Some old-time beliefs about what pollen can do follow (please remember, these are home remedies, not scientifically proven cures!):

Combine pollen and kelp for those with low blood pressure, fainting and general weakness.

An application of pollen can soothe and begin the healing process for skin blemishes.

For faster healing, sprinkle pollen that has been mixed with flour on open sores and burns.

Scandinavians mix honey, pollen and oil from fish liver. This is used on skin blemishes.

Sipping honey and pollen together is an old European remedy for an irritated throat.

For bronchial problems, Europeans apply a honey and pollen poultice to the throat.

It has been said that drinking milk mixed with honey and pollen will produce a voice with golden tones.

Pollen and lemon juice in boiled water make a tea for soothing a sore throat. This has been used for lung problems, too.

An old New England remedy for sleeplessness is made by combining 2 tablespoons honey, 1 teaspoon pollen, 1 teaspoon apple cider vinegar and 3/4 cup hot water. This sleep tonic works best if taken while it is warm.

For extra energy and vitality, eat honey and pollen with a little ginseng in it.

Constipation can be relieved by eating honey spread on whole wheat bread and sprinkled with pollen.

A tablespoon of honey, with a little pollen mixed in, is an old time diuretic.

Ease an aching throat by gargling with a tea made of boiled rose hips and pollen, sweetened with honey.

For a special treat, use pollen in your favorite facial cleanser. Or soak a couple of teaspoons of pollen in 1/3 cup buttermilk and wipe it on the face. Let the face soak a bit, then rinse gently in cool water.

Add a small dash of pollen to shampoo for healthy, shiny hair.

An old remedy for dandruff is made from equal parts vinegar and water, with a sprinkle of pollen added to it. Just rub it on the scalp and shampoo as usual.

Soak tired feet in warm water to which a teaspoon of pollen and 1/3 cup apple cider vinegar have been added. They will soon be revitalized!

Propolis – Is it a Wonder Cure?

Propolis is a resinous substance that can be found around leaf buds and on the bark of trees. Honeybees gather it to patch holes in the hive and to use as a protective film around anything that dies in the hive.

Several scientific tests have just been completed on the healing properties of Propolis. Some researchers are claiming it is a new wonder remedy!

Propolis is the sticky sap-like stuff deciduous and conifer trees secrete when they are damaged. It seals the injury and protects trees from disease. Bees gather it and use it as hive cement, and maybe, to disinfect bees as they come into the hive.

This sticky, medium-brown resin has a vanilla sort of smell, much like new-mown hay. It is being tested as a healing treatment for stomach ulcers and as an antiviral agent.

Propolis is thought to promote healing by stimulating the immune system. It has been shown to have more antibacterial activity than penicillin!

In Russia, it is mixed with honey and fed to patients before surgery to guard against infection.

Some chew propolis, like gum, as a treatment for gum disease.

It is said that propolis and honey make a salve for promoting the healing of bruises.

Propolis is used in many creams for soothing dermatitis caused by both bacteria and fungus. It also reduces mold growth.

Tradition says Italian violin makers of long ago used propolis in their secret varnish recipes. It was supposed to be part of the process that developed the wondrous tone of those famous old violins.

Royal Jelly

Brood food, bee milk, royal jelly – these are all names for the food nurse bees make. It is excreted from the pharyngeal glands in their heads after they have eaten lots of pollen.

Royal jelly is rich in proteins and vitamins. It contains 18 amino acids and has gamma globulin for fighting infection. In 6 days it can multiply a larva's weight 1,500 times.

Queen bees are very fertile and live much longer than other bees. This is because they eat royal jelly. It is a thick, white, milky liquid. Only nurse bees make it.

Royal jelly is a potent substance. Some say it is an elixir of youth, rejuvenating to humans and good for treating disease. Supposedly, it is a mood enhancer, an aphrodisiac and a wrinkle remover.

Emotional problems, senility, insomnia, eczema and upset stomachs are said to respond to royal jelly.

Beeswax
The wax that is naturally formed inside the hive is called beeswax. It is mostly used as a foundation for the bees' hive in the formation of honeycombs.

As a general rule, about it takes about 10 pounds of honey to form a single pound of beeswax.

Beeswax is more expensive than honey and has many practical uses:

- Madame Tussaud's wax museum uses 75% pure beeswax for its figures because it makes wax skin seem translucent.

- Dentists use it for impressions

- Others use hot wax treatments to comfort arthritic hands and feet.

- Beeswax is used with zinc and castor oil in ointments for diaper rash and it is the base of lipstick. (Add turpentine and it is furniture polish)

- Sail makers, cobblers and tailors have long waxed thread to add strength and durability. Ropes are treated with wax to make them last longer, too.

- As a protective coating for aging cheeses

- Beeswax is used in making fine candles

- Musicians are familiar with beeswax that can go into making a covering on tambourines or rosin for string instruments.

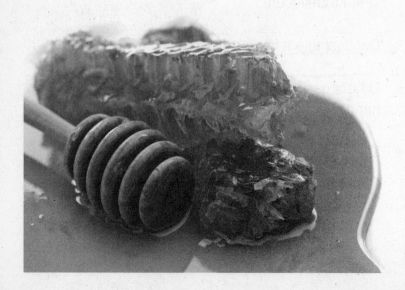

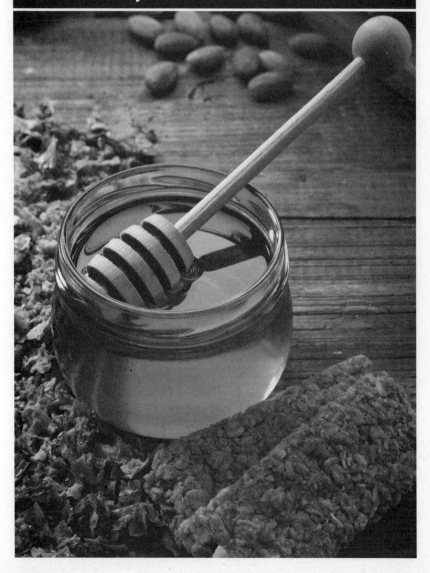

CHAPTER SIX
Honey Home Remedies

Honey's healing properties have been well documented and established in the research community. While you and I probably won't be preserving corneas in honey solutions for transplant patients any time soon, we can look at various home remedies using honey that have been passed down for generations.

Down through countless ages honey has been regarded with awe and wonder. In some Mediterranean communities honey was even used, in place of gold or silver, as money. Honey has not only been considered a sacred food, fit for feeding deities, it has been part of the folk medicine of nearly every culture on the planet.

Rameses III, Pharaoh of Egypt, felt honey was so important to the people he supplied honey to his priests for festivals. The Greek philosopher Pythagoras linked his long life to honey. Mohammed is reported to have used honey for healing. The Talmud recommends honey for gout, heart trouble and healing wounds in man and beast.

Honey is nature's original all-purpose dressing for skin ailments. Traditionally, honey has been part of remedies for respiratory tract afflictions such as coughs, colds, bronchitis and asthma.

This chapter takes a look at many of the most popular, and some seldom heard of, honey home remedies that have been passed down through generations. Remember, many of these are folk remedies, not necessarily scientifically proven cures. It is for you, the reader to judge how much use they are to your specific situation. What works for one person, may not work for you.

When using honey externally as a topical salve, it is best to use honey which is as raw, or unprocessed and as unrefined, as possible. It is with this honey that one may receive the greatest healing benefit. The more processing honey undergoes, and the more heat that is used in the processing, the greater the degradation that takes place. Greater degradation translates into less useful honey when it comes to home remedy use.

For honey that is going to be used externally, remember to keep it separated from kitchen honey as a precaution. You can even store this honey in your medicine cabinet or label it with a handwritten label for easy identification.

For honey taken internally, again, honey that is more pure retains more of its vitamins, minerals and useful enzymes. Also, while honey can certainly be used in warm teas or heated in sauces, keep in mind that excessive heat is the enemy. Too much heat can destroy the best parts about honey, rendering its medicinal qualities somewhat useless.

And please remember: when using honey as a natural home remedy, care must be taken to be sure the honey has not gotten too old for proper use, or has harmful bacteria which could make an open cut or wound become infected. And take caution to never give honey to infants younger than one year of age.

Coughs, Colds and Throat Tickles

Honey has long been used to increase the healing ability of other foods. A syrup to ease coughs and irritable throats can be produced by spreading honey on these curative foods, waiting a few hours, then drawing off the syrup that forms. To prepare: cut open a turnip, garlic clove, radish, onion or lemon. Spread a thin coating of honey over the cut side of the food. In a few hours an effective cough syrup will have formed.

Many herbs can be mixed into honey to make powerful cough suppressors. Make herb-honey cough remedies by mincing 1/4 teaspoon herb into 1/2 cup honey. Let stand for several hours before feeding very small amounts. Some herbs to use this way include: fennel, anise, horehound and thyme.

Each day, chew a piece of honeycomb made by bees native to your specific area. You will be much less troubled by ailments of the breathing tract and lungs.

Try making your own honey lollipops to bring relief to a troubling sore throat. These are great for children who can suck on the lollipops as often as needed:

Honey Lollipops
1/3 cup honey
1 cup sugar
3 T light corn syrup
1 T water
Candy sticks

1. Line a cookie sheet or tray with wax paper.
2. In a heavy pan, add honey, sugar, corn syrup and water. Cook over medium heat until mixture is dissolved and combined.
3. Continue cooking until mixture has reached 300°F when checked with a candy thermometer.
4. Pour small dollops of candy solution onto wax paper (or use a candy mold). Quickly add candy sticks making sure honey solution encompasses the sticks.
5. Allow to cool completely, about 20 minutes.
6. Gently peel back wax paper from lollipops. Wrap in plastic or additional wax paper and store in a cool, dry place until ready to use.

Quiet a stubborn cough by swallowing small amounts of well-ripened honey. Allow this honey to ease down the throat slowly, coating the throat as it goes down.

For a nagging cough before bedtime, try a teaspoon or two of honey to ease the coughing and allow for restful sleep.

For a honey concoction to sip on throughout the day, combine a cup of honey with a few tablespoons of lemon juice. Sip throughout the day to bring relief to an aching sore throat.

To clear a stuffy head, combine a tablespoon or two of honey in a basin with hot water. Place a towel over the basin with your head beneath and inhale some of the warm vapor.

Sweetened radish juice, to treat coughs and hoarseness, is prepared by scooping out the middle of a radish and filling it with honey. In a couple of hours the cavity will be filled with juice.

To relive the pain of a sore throat, gargle with a glass of warm water with a tablespoon of dark honey stirred into it. For even more healing power, add a teaspoon of lemon juice.

Stir one tablespoon of honey into warm lemon tea to calm a nagging cough.

Honey made from sunflowers is a good aid in reducing fevers. Use it in tea or take by the spoonful.

Arthritis and Joint Pain

Soothe the discomfort of arthritis and rheumatism by eating a wee bit of honey with each meal.

Relieve the pain of arthritis and rheumatism by applying a warm honey-pack. To prepare, heat 1 cup honey and 1 cup water until nicely warm. Wring out a soft cloth in this mixture and apply to the hurting joint.

Many beekeepers believe they are protected from rheumatism and arthritis because of the frequent bee stings they get.

When gout troubles you, apply a warm honey compress. It will soothe the pain.

Ease the discomfort of arthritis or rheumatism by sipping a cup of warm willow tea, sweetened with honey, before retiring for the evening.

A daily dose of lavender honey is good for arthritis sufferers.

Mix a tablespoon or two of honey with equal parts apple cider vinegar into a glass of warm water to bring relief to aching joint pain.

To relieve the joint pain of arthritis and rheumatism, allow a honeybee to sting the afflicted area. Use a glass jar to catch a foraging bee as it leaves the hive in the morning. It will be healthy and vigorous. Put the jar over the hurting joint and gently shake until the bee stings.

Ease arthritis and joint pain with this elixir to drink daily. In a mug of warm water, mix a tablespoon or two each of honey and apple cider vinegar.

Ease the pain of leg cramps by swallowing 2 teaspoons apple cider vinegar sweetened with a teaspoon of honey every night.

Digestion and Laxatives

Strengthen the constitution of one who has a weak digestive system by feeding them honey on a regular basis.

A dab of honey makes a good digestive aid for one who has weak kidneys.

To combat an upset stomach or digestive tract, try mixing a tablespoon of honey and a tablespoon of apple cider vinegar into a glass of fruit juice or warm tea.

For upset stomach or vomiting, slowly take a swallow or two of honey throughout the day.

A few spoonfuls of fresh from-the-hive honey is a gentle, effective laxative.

Problems with constipation? Try a tablespoon of honey, three times a day as a gentle, natural laxative.

New honey is the best kind to use as a laxative.

Aid indigestion and prevent heart and kidney problems by sipping tea made of boiled parsley and honey.

Serve small amounts of honey to one suffering from diarrhea. It helps prevent dehydration.

Immune and Body
Boost your body's weak immune system with a sip of warm honey tea. For the most part, the darker the amber color of the honey, the higher in antioxidant properties the honey contains. Two or three teaspoons of honey in a cup of tea will do.

Those deficient in essential minerals and vitamins can increase their general health by eating a small piece of honey, in the comb, each day.

Allergies

Take a teaspoon of honey made by bees from your own locality with each meal. It will help to relieve hay fever symptoms.

To prevent hay fever, chew on a piece of honeycomb from a local hive. Do this twice a day for several weeks before the hay fever season begins. Also, eat 1 teaspoon of honey with each meal.

Chewing on a honeycomb several times a day can help strengthen the overall immune system for people suffering from allergies or asthma.

Respiratory Ailments and Infections

Eucalyptus, lavender and pine honey are best for respiratory infections.

Relieve asthmatic symptoms with a spoonful of honey sprinkled with cinnamon. This works best when taken just before bedtime each night.

For breathing troubles, try to slowly sip on a cup of warm tea sweetened liberally with honey.

Make a soothing vapor mist of warm water, vinegar and a splash of honey.

Try a warm tea made from honey, lemon juice and ginger to break up chest congestion and give easier breathing.

Cuts, Scrapes and Open Wounds

Raw honey, since it has not gone through the refining process which can destroy much of honey's antibacterial and antimicrobial benefits and is still in its most pure form, works best for healing cuts, scrapes and as a treatment for open wounds.

Wipe down a new injury 3 times a day with honey and it will not become infected.

Wipe down an old injury 5 times a day with honey and it will soon begin to heal.

Cuts and scrapes heal faster and are less likely to become infected if bathed in a lotion made of equal parts honey and cod liver oil. This is also good for improving the complexion.

Gently warm 1/4 cup light colored beeswax with 1 cup strained honey. Stir well and then allow to cool to room temperature. Makes a wonderfully healing salve for open sores that refuse to heal.

Mix 1/3 cup honey and 2/3 cup lard together for a good ointment for cuts and other injuries.

For cuts, scrapes or wounds, apply about a tablespoon of honey onto a 2" x 2" gauze pad and secure over the affected area. Do not allow bandage to become dry, changing the bandage and honey a couple of times throughout the day.

Use a little dab of honey on a large adhesive bandage. Change the dressing several times a day to promote rapid healing.

Bandages or gauze dampened with honey make a soothing treatment for varicose ulcers.

Bites and Boils

Use a moist paste made up of honey and flour on insect bites to help heal the wound in faster time.

Soak a small piece of horseradish overnight in 1/2 cup honey. Use as a healing bath for abscesses and boils.

Take the pain from a bee sting or the itch from a mosquito bite by covering them with honey.

Treat a fresh bee sting by dabbing a little fresh honey on the wound as soon as you are stung. Repeat as often as needed for healing relief.

Burns

Honey can be used to ease the pain of summer sunburns. Just use your fingers full of honey, slightly moistened with water to help glide painlessly over sunburns, to ease discomfort. Some studies show sunburn can heal up to 3 or 4 days faster with honey, than without.

Use the same honey treatment on minor burns from scalding.

Burns to the fingers or hands can be treated by gently applying honey to the affected area.

For burned areas, apply a generous amount of raw honey to a sterile bandage and cover the burned area, securing with tape. Change this dressing several times a day to help promote rapid healing. Dressing should not become dry. If it does, the dressing needs changed more often.

Raw honey is best for burns, as this honey has not been heat processed which can destroy most of it healing properties.

For large or deep burns, be careful not to introduce bacteria into the burn that could be lingering in some types of honey. Always consult your physician if you are concerned about whether honey can be beneficial to a burn.

Fatigue
Stamina and endurance may be increased by eating a little honey every day.

Extreme fatigue and apathy may be relieved by taking a tablespoon of honey with the noon meal.

Some say a spoonful of equal parts honey and cinnamon can bring relief to feelings of fatigue.

A drink of 2 parts honey to 1 part cinnamon mixed in a glass of water can bring relief from fatigue.

Sweet Sleep: Battling Insomnia
To ensure a good night's sleep, sip on a glass of warm milk to which a spoonful of honey has been added.

Prevent nighttime leg cramps that keep a body from its nightly rest by taking a teaspoonful of honey with each meal. Also helps to stop twitches and jerks of eyelids and lips.

Soothe nighttime leg cramps by taking 1 teaspoon clover honey at bedtime.

A spoonful of honey taken 30 – 40 minutes before bedtime will ensure sweet dreams and a good night's sleep.

Children and Babies*
A spoonful of honey at bedtime will keep a child from wetting the bed.

A glass of barley water with a tablespoon of honey in it makes a good health drink for youngsters.

Little ones thrive if fed with a mixture of buttermilk and honey.

Soothe a sore diaper rash bottom with a coating of honey.

Skin, Hands and Nails
A little horseradish juice stirred into some honey will reduce flaking in skin irritations.

Grate 1/2 teaspoon fresh horseradish into 1/4 cup honey and apply to toenails that are infested with fungus. It will hurry along the healing process. This is also good for any sore that does not heal quickly.

Pat honey, fresh from the comb, on a sunburn to ease the sting. It will hasten healing, lighten the pain, and prevent scarring. Wet the fingers before using them to apply honey and it will slide on much smoother.

Mix equal parts honey and olive oil for a soothing lotion for dry skin.

Use a quick application of honey as a moisture barrier for dry, cracked and healing skin.

Soak the face in honey each evening for a youthful, wrinkle free complexion.

Dry, chapped hands may be healed by rubbing them with honey each morning and evening. Leave on for 3 minutes, rinse and dry thoroughly.

Prevent wrinkles and tiny age lines by soaking the face each morning in 1 tablespoon heavy cream, mixed with 1 teaspoon honey. Rinse off with cool water and pat the skin dry.

Honey holds moisture, so it is good for moisturizing the skin. It also draws dirt from pores, leaving the skin fresh, clean and youthful looking.

Fight cold sores by dabbing them every few hours with undiluted honey. Dark honey is best.

Stir 2 tablespoons honey into a quart of warm water and use to rinse the face. Skin will look young and healthy and have a rosy glow.

Use a milk bath and honey soak for luxurious skin during the dry winter months.

Treat your skin to a gentle facial mask. Apply honey directly to the face and neck, allowing it to dry completely. This should take about 15 to 20 minutes. Rinse clean with warm water and gently pat dry.

Make your own honey facial scrub. Combine one tablespoon honey with two teaspoons lemon juice. Add about a tablespoon of sugar and incorporate well. Use scrub to exfoliate facial skin for a smooth, refreshed appearance.

Because honey is such an effective moisturizer and skin softener, it is a natural for preparing facials. One of the best is made by combining 1 egg yolk, 1 tablespoon honey and 1 tablespoon oatmeal. Pat on and let dry, then rinse with lots of clear water.

Honey is a wonderful moisturizer for those with sensitive skin. Simply dab your fingers in honey, then into a bit of cool water to make honey glide over the skin effortlessly. Rinse and gently pat dry.

A very good way to soften and clean the skin is to wipe it down with equal parts of honey and yogurt.

Dabbing a few dots of honey on stubborn acne can help give a clear complexion.

Next time you find yourself with dry, chapped lips, reach for some honey! A thin layer of honey on the lips can bring soothing relief.

Cleanse the face by covering it with a blend of 1 teaspoon honey and 1 tablespoon either sweet or sour cream. Rinse off with cool water.

Add about a half a cup of honey to warm bath water for an all over skin softener.

Hair and More

Fight hair loss, and improve the texture of remaining hair, by rubbing 1 tablespoon honey, 1 tablespoon vodka and 1 teaspoon onion juice on the head each evening.

Want a new, natural way to combat dandruff? Combine honey with a dab of olive oil to form a soft gel. Rub into the scalp and allow to remain about 20 minutes. Shampoo out, leaving your hair and scalp free from dry dandruff flakes.

Encourage new hair to grow on a bald head by rubbing the head with a cut onion. Then pat on a covering of honey and let set overnight. Rinse off with warm water in the morning.

Try a new conditioning rinse to leave your hair shiny. In a bottle or jar, mix three or four cups of warm water with a teaspoon of honey and a tablespoon of lemon juice. Use as a final hair rinse, leaving in the hair, at the end of your bath or shower.

Mix 1 tablespoon honey with 1 cup warm water. It makes an exceptional rinse for the hair.

Miscellaneous

Relieve the discomfort of an overly dry mouth by gargling with honey-water. To prepare, add 1/4 cup honey to one quart water. Mix well and gargle with a small amount. Repeat as needed.

For quick relief from an aching tooth, make a paste by combining 1 teaspoon honey with 1/4 teaspoon cinnamon. Apply directly to affected tooth as necessary.

Battling a sinus infection? Try a glass of warm tea with a tablespoon of honey mixed in with an equal tablespoon of apple cider vinegar.

Honey can make a wonderful, antibacterial mouthwash. Just mix a few teaspoons of honey into a glass of warm water, gargle and rinse.

Need a solution for bad breath? Try gargling with a warm water solution of 1 tablespoon of honey mixed with a half teaspoon cinnamon for fresh breath and a clean mouth.

To bring relief from a headache, stir a tablespoon of honey into a glass of water and drink.

Honey and warm water can help treat pink eye or conjunctivitis.

A tea made of sage and honey is said to ease the pain of shingles. Steep about a cup of fresh sage in a quart of water for an hour. Sweeten with 1 cup honey and take 1 teaspoon each hour.

Replacing white table sugar with honey can be beneficial for heart patients.

Irritated by hiccups? Try consuming very small amounts of honey mixed with ginger every 20 minutes for relief.

Better Health

A healthy restorative for those who have been ill can be made by mixing honey, corn meal and bananas.

Give new energy to one who is anemic by serving them buckwheat honey every day.

Old honey is the best kind to use for healing tonics; use newer honey for dressings on open wounds, cuts and scrapes.

Honey, parsley seeds and snails (shells and all) may be ground together for a nostrum that is said to discourage the body from making gallstones.

The best honey to eat for good eyesight is made from the blossoms of the thyme plant.

Strengthen weak and afflicted lungs by sipping daily on water with a little honey stirred in.

*NEVER feed honey to a child under 1 year of age. Some honeys may contain botulism spores which can be extremely dangerous to babies under one year of age.

Just A Few More
Make any healing remedy more potent by taking a little honey and water with it.

For a natural healing remedy for goiter, try crushing an onion and mixing with equal parts honey and olive oil.

Lose weight by ending each meal with a teaspoon of honey. It replaces higher calorie desserts and leaves the body feeling full and satisfied.

A teaspoon of honey in a glass of water, 30 minutes before each meal, will help restrain the over robust appetite.

Improve general health by drinking a tonic made by simmering chopped rose petals in honey.

Drive worms from the body with a tonic made by boiling a handful of rue, 1 cup wine, and 1 cup honey. Take a couple of spoonfuls before each meal.

The best honey for treating urinary tract infections and anemia is made from heather blossoms.

Warmed honey makes a wonderful massage lotion for aching bodies. Not only can this loosen tight and sore muscles, but will leave the skin feeling soft, supple and refreshed as well.

It is said that a teaspoon or two of honey is a natural libido enhancer.

Sweet Friendships

Welcome a new member to the family by sharing a dish made of 1 cup curds, 1 cup honey and 1 cup butter, well mixed together. This will cause the relationship to be long, peaceful and sweet. (Dry cottage cheese may be substituted for the curds.)

Seal a new friendship by sharing milk sweetened with honey. It will guarantee that only sweet words will pass between the friends.

An enduring relationship is assured if two people share some freshly baked bread which has been spread with equal parts butter and honey.

Eat some honey each day to have a strong heart and a quick mind well into old age.

Ensure a happy and prosperous year by eating rice sweetened with honey on New Year's Day.

To ensure lasting friendships and good relations with neighbors, serve them a bit of heavy cream, sweetened with honey. May be sipped from a small glass or served as a spread on warm bread.

Tonics and Good Fortune

For nearly instant energy, eat a tablespoon of honey. This is a good restorative after exercise or other exertion.

Each day will be happy and profitable if it begins with a dose of honey, spread on freshly baked bread.

Relieve the symptoms of a hangover by taking 1 teaspoon honey and 1 full glass of water each hour.

Orange blossom honey is soothing to those with nervous afflictions.

Honey Around the Home

To keep the water in a car radiator from freezing, add honey to it. It makes a cheap antifreeze solution.

Twigs for tree grafts can be preserved and made more vigorous by soaking them in honey.

Sprinkle the foundation stones of a new home with honey. This will guarantee that those who live there will live long, happy lives.

Gather honey in the spring for high flavor and delightful aroma.

Gather honey in the fall to use for cooking and healing remedies.

To keep seeds from deteriorating, store them in a glass jar filled with honey.

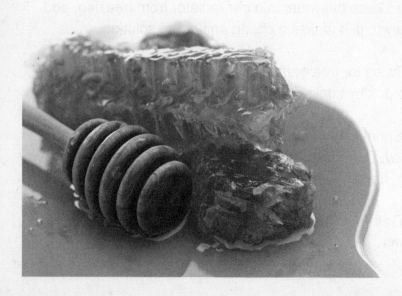

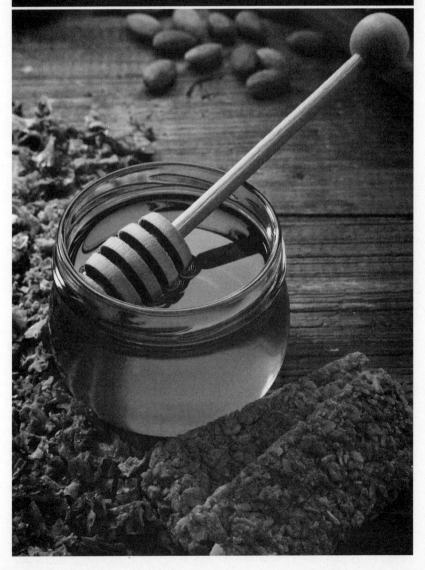

CHAPTER SEVEN
Honey & Vinegar

Honey and apple cider vinegar* are an age-old combination for a healthy body and mind. Honey brings a sweet dose of nearly instant energy and vinegar supplies a tart complement. Both are natural storehouses of amino acids, healthful enzymes and trace minerals.

Down through the ages many have claimed that when these two foods are combined they are a nearly magical elixir for good health. This chapter deals with the special mixing of these two ingredients to form all new remedies for common ailments.

Why vinegar? Vinegar has been credited with possessing a surprising number of health-promoting qualities. Many researchers believe this is because of its unique combination of ingredients. It contains bits of proteins, fiber and carbohydrates, calcium, iron, vitamins and minerals, just to name a few. It is because of these special traits that make vinegar a natural health paring with honey.

Now, they may not be a cure-all for every ailment of mankind, but they do supply a host of nutrients needed for good health. And, just how all the good things in both honey and apple cider vinegar work together inside the body is not completely understood, even today.

*You may wish to reference The Vinegar Book in the back of this volume for more information on more ways vinegar can be used both as a home remedy and around the house.

On the pages which follow are some of the best of the many ways honey and apple cider vinegar have been used together for health and well-being. Because old-time remedies are handed down from generation to generation, they have a way of evolving with the years. Still, they have a consistent theme: some small amount of sweet golden honey, combined with tangy apple cider vinegar, is a very special remedy for whatever ails most anyone! (Please remember, these are folk remedies, not scientifically proven cures!):

Coughs, Colds and Sore Throats
Boil a cutup lemon in 1 cup apple cider vinegar until the lemon is soft and mushy. Mash the lemon up as much as possible, then strain. Add enough honey to make 1 cup liquid (about 1/2 cup honey will be needed). Take 1 teaspoon of this syrup whenever a cough or the pain of a sore throat becomes troublesome.

The very best cough suppressor is made by combining honey, garlic and apple cider vinegar. To make, peel 10 garlic cloves and cook them in 1 cup apple cider vinegar until they are soft and mushy. Mash well and stir into 1 cup honey. Keep this wondrous cough remedy in a tightly covered jar. Shake well before each use. A single teaspoonful, taken as needed, will bring surprising results.

Chop up a peeled potato and boil it in 1 cup water, to which 1/4 cup apple cider vinegar has been added. When the potato is soft, mash it into the liquid and stir in 1/4 cup clover honey. A tablespoon of this mixture, every half hour, will soon relieve a troublesome cough.

Relieve a nagging cough by taking 1 teaspoon of the following, each hour. Heat 1/2 cup olive oil with 3 tablespoons apple cider vinegar. When very warm, remove from heat and add 1 cup honey. Mix well.

Coughs and sore throats can be eased by taking small spoonfuls of honey which has been fortified with apple cider vinegar and hot pepper. To prepare, mix 1/3 cup clover honey with 1/4 cup vinegar. When the honey is dissolved, add 1 teaspoon hot-red pepper.

A honey-baked beet can go a long way toward ending a bothersome cough. To prepare, split a large beet in half and scoop out a small hollow in the middle of each half. Fill the hole in the beet halves with honey, cover, and bake until the beet is tender. Scoop the soft beet out of the peeling and mash 1 tablespoon apple cider vinegar into it. (May be served with a dab of sour cream.)

For a quick and easy remedy to treat sore throats, heat 1/4 cup apple cider vinegar and 1 teaspoon grated onion in the microwave. Stir the hot mixture into 2/3 cup honey. Take a teaspoon before each meal and at bedtime.

To relieve a sore throat, gargle with a glass of warm water to which 1 teaspoon honey and 1 teaspoon apple cider vinegar have been added. This helps because honey is a mild sedative and pain killer, and both honey and apple cider vinegar have antiseptic qualities.

Inside the Body and Out

Relieve the pain of arthritis, rheumatism and other aches and pains by applying a warm honey-pack to the afflicted area. To prepare, heat 1 cup honey and 3/4 cup apple cider vinegar until nicely warm. Soak a soft cloth in this mixture, squeeze out the excess liquid, and drape it over the place that hurts.

Soothe a troubled stomach by slowly sipping a glass of warm water with 1 tablespoon honey and 1 tablespoon apple cider vinegar added to it.

Insomnia may be banished by using a concoction of 1 cup honey and 2 tablespoons apple cider vinegar. Mix it up and keep it at bedside. Swallow a teaspoon of this sleep inducing elixir once every hour you are awake in the night.

Encourage good general health and fight illness by beginning each day with this special oatmeal. Prepare by boiling a serving of oatmeal in water to which a teaspoon of apple cider vinegar has been added. Serve with 1 tablespoon honey dribbled across the top.

Improve facial skin with this 10 minute cleansing treatment. Mix 1 tablespoon honey, 1 teaspoon olive oil and 1 egg yolk. Pat onto the face and neck. After 10 minutes rinse in cool water and gently dry.

Renew oily skin and make it glow with good health by rinsing it daily with equal parts honey and apple cider vinegar.

Use 1 tablespoon honey, 1 teaspoon apple cider vinegar and 1 egg white to tighten sagging skin. Remove after 10 minutes by rinsing in cool water.

Honey Vinegar
Mead, a mildly alcoholic drink made when water and honey ferment, was a staple in the Old English diet. Just as cider ferments into apple cider vinegar, mead ferments into honey vinegar.

Honey vinegar can be used much in the same ways as apple cider vinegar (or any other vinegar). In old-time England a very special healing potion, called oxymel, was made by combining fresh honey and honey vinegar.

Prepare oxymel by adding fresh honey, sea salt and newly caught rainwater to honey vinegar. The uses for this special elixir are countless.

Some ways oxymel was used in England follow:

Sip on oxymel to relieve pain and inflammation of the throat.

Drink oxymel and you will clear up troubles of the ears.

Rheumatic disorders will be relieved by taking oxymel.

Back pain may be lightened by drinking well made oxymel.

Treat gout by sipping regularly on oxymel.

Rub oxymel on sore joints to relieve the aches and pains of old age.

Use newly made oxymel as the liquid for preparing vegetables and the family will stay healthy and not suffer from diseases of the digestive system.

A good remedy for insomnia is a daily dose of oxymel.

Relieve constipation by eating a nice helping of oxymel each day.

Apply oxymel to sore joints and aches and pains will disappear.

Pickled Honey Delights
Apicius, an ancient Roman food authority, described one of his country folks' favorite foods, pickled turnips. They were preserved in vinegar, sweetened with honey, and flavored with lots of myrtle berries.

Vinegar, sweetened with honey and enlivened with spices, is good for pickling a variety of fruits and for making relish.

Make fruit pickles by simmering cut pieces in a spicy honey and vinegar syrup. Try peaches, pears, plums or melon rinds.

A few grape leaves added to fruit pickles will keep the fruit from becoming mushy.

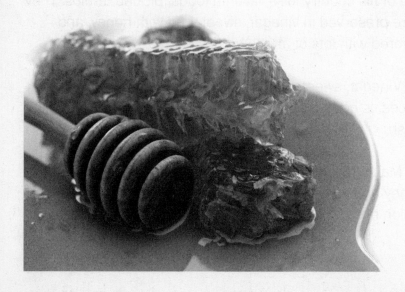

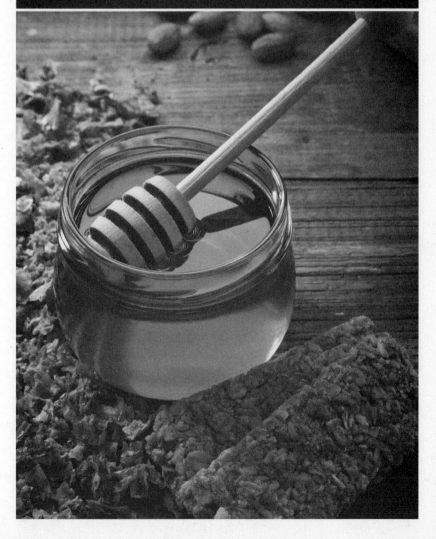

CHAPTER EIGHT
Honey Rich
Foods & Drinks

Honey is one of our most treasured links with ancient mankind. Honey eating predates bread, milk and cereals. In olden times, things were not routinely sweet, so folks treasured sweetness as a rare and valuable commodity; a special treat.

Sugarcane's use dates back to the 1300s in India, and was not planted in Southern Europe until 100 years later. Then, it was another 100 years before it became widely available in Northern Europe. Before this time, honey was about the only sweetener most folks had.

We have come a long way since the time when an Egyptian bridegroom was expected to promise his bride a jar of honey for each month of the year. Today, honey can be an expensive food for the most discriminating of palates or a natural food for those who seek to replace nutritionally empty foods with more natural ones.

Whatever your reason for choosing honey as a sweetener, you are joining generations of those who have come to appreciate its golden goodness.

Choose the Right Honey
There is more to honey than just sweetness. It adds its own unique flavor to dishes and makes a subtle difference in the texture and color of foods. Depending upon the variety chosen, honey's flavor can be a delicate hint of richness or a robust flavor change. These differences should be taken into account when choosing which honey to pare with different foods.

Clover honey is a good choice for most cooking needs. Its mild flavor easily adaptable to most recipes. Use delicate flavors, like orange blossom and thyme for spreads, where their fine flavors can be appreciated. Use strong honeys, like wild flower and buckwheat in cookies, gingerbread and highly spiced foods.

When buying honey in the comb, look for an even, light color. While some honeycomb can be naturally dark, it is more likely that a dark color occurs because it is old or has been exposed to high temperatures.

Honey which has separated may be spoiled. This only happens if the water content is extremely high, and usually means the honey was diluted with water or less costly corn syrup. One can frequently find this when using USDA labeled "substandard" grades of honey.

Cooking with Honey
When honey is substituted for granulated sugar in recipes, amounts must be adjusted slightly. Generally, about half the sugar in a recipe can be replaced with honey without seriously affecting the action of leavening ingredients.

Honey is about twice as sweet as sugar, and contains about 20% water. So, replace each 1/2 cup of sugar with about 1/4 cup honey, and reduce the total liquid in each recipe by about a tablespoon or two. This will prevent the food from becoming too mushy.

When a baked recipe has had part of its sugar replaced with honey, it is usually a good idea to cook it at a temperature which is about 25 degrees lower than usual. This will keep the baked good from browning too soon, producing a more desired end result.

Because honey is hygroscopic, meaning it can absorb moisture that is found in the air, it helps keep cakes and breads moist for a longer length of time.

Replacing sugar with honey can help cut the number of calories in the diet. There are 78 calories in two tablespoons of sugar and 126 calories in two tablespoons of honey. Since honey has twice the sweetening power of sugar, it is only necessary to use half as much. So, 78 calories of sugar can be replaced with 63 calories of honey. That is about a 20% savings in calories.

Make measuring honey easy by first warming it. Rinsing utensils in warm water helps, too. When using honey in recipes that also require oil, measure out the oil first, leaving the measuring cup or spoon slickly coated for the honey. This will allow the honey to fall out of the measuring utensil more effortlessly.

Honey which has become crystallized can be liquefied by gently warming it. A few seconds in a microwave oven will do this. Or, set the honey in a pan of warm water for a few minutes, and gently swirl it around. This should bring honey back to its original liquid state quite easily.

Honey-Rich Foods

With the many amazing ways honey is good for the human body, incorporating this wonderful syrup into an everyday healthy diet is both simple and delicious. Many foods are not nearly as good if sweetened with anything other than the liquid gold we call honey.

Some of the most popular honey enhanced foods include:

- Honeyed salad dressings, made with mustard, oil, vinegar or lemon juice and herbs.

- Roast duck or chicken, crusted with tarragon, ginger or orange sauce

- Honeyed leeks, onions or garlic are caramelized delights that deliver lots of healing nutrients.

- Fish, lamb, or pork roast with a honey and lemon topping.

- Honey drizzled over fresh fruit chunks then sprinkled with raisins.

- Honey glazed apples, dotted with raisins.

- Cabbage cooked with honey and caraway seeds.

- Honey as a topping for ice cream or served warm over baked goods and other desserts.

- Dijon, the honey-mustard sauce made of apple cider vinegar, mustard, wine, honey, lemon juice, onion, garlic and spices.

- Gingerbread, a delightful bouquet of baked spices, set off by generous amounts of honey.

- Nearly any recipe which includes nuts is enhanced by honey. The honey-nut association goes back to some of the most ancient recipes.

- Honey's unique taste goes well with the gentle flavor of eggs and dairy products like milk, sweet or sour cream and yogurt.

- Honey as a basting sauce or marinade for grilled chicken or a steaks.

- Used as a base sauce for oriental stir fry dishes.

- Baklava, torrone or other Mediterranean desserts are known for their delicious honey coatings.

When honey is used in a sauce, it should be added at the very end of the cooking process. The heat of cooking can ruin the flavor and gentle fragrance of light, delicate honeys.

In baked good, such as breads, add honey early in the mixing process so the enzymes in it can act on other ingredients before the heat of baking kills them. For example, when using honey as the active ingredient with yeast breads, make certain to allow enough time for the honey to produce a reaction with yeast before baking the bread.

Traditional English breakfast porridge was made of a variety of chopped fruits, such as oranges, apples, blackberries and raisins and nuts such as walnuts. The mixture was drizzled with honey and lemon juice, mixed with oatmeal, and served with either milk or cream.

Sweet Treats

Honey is used as the basis for candy in countries all across the world. Many recipes begin with a fondant-type mixture of sugar, honey and water. This liquid is boiled until it reaches the soft ball stage, then stirred or kneaded until smooth and light in color.

These smooth, fondant candies are used to stuff dates or figs, or formed into small balls wrapped around pieces of fruits or nuts. Fondant can also be dipped into a variety of coverings, including chocolate.

When fondant has nuts or fruits mixed into it, it is usually called a nougat. When making various nougats, the liquid is usually boiled to the hard ball stage (250° - 266°) and stirred into beaten egg whites. These two types of honey-sweetened candy are the basis for:

- Italy's torrone, which has egg whites, candied fruit, toasted almonds and hazelnuts kneaded into it.

- Spain's turron, made with toasted almonds and a little flour.

- France's nougat, which adds egg whites, almonds and cherries.

- Turkey and Greece's halvah, made by adding sesame oil, ground nuts, farina, ground cloves and cinnamon.

All of these are wrapped in edible rice paper, and need to be kept tightly covered, as the honey will cause them to attract moisture from the air.

When combining honey and sugar for fondants and nougats, the greater the proportion of sugar, the firmer the final product will be. A high proportion of honey keeps the final candy soft and creamy.

In addition to boiling it with sugar, honey is encouraged to "set up" by adding varying amounts of flour, ground nuts or sesame seeds. Other sweet treats which are especially good when made with honey include:

- Divinity, made with beaten egg whites, like a nougat.

- Taffy, made with honey, water, sugar and a splash of vinegar is "pulled" while warm, rather than beaten.

- Peanut brittle, a mixture of honey, sugar, water and butter, boiled until it is very concentrated and poured over nuts.

Honey Vinegars

Honey and vinegar may, at first glance, seem like an odd paring. But the truth is, the sweetness of golden honey pared with the acidity of vinegar makes for a truly wonderful and delicious accompaniment.

For some of the best results, try using apple cider vinegar. The tartness of the apples works hand in hand with the sweet flow of honey. For a more daring approach, why not try some of the flavored and fortified vinegars offered in gourmet shops. Or better yet, try making your own!

Sweet peach and honey vinegar is particularly delicious for summer salads. Simmer 3 cups cut-up peaches in a quart of apple cider vinegar for about 20 minutes. Strain, add 1/4 cup mild honey and put in a plastic container with a tight-fitting lid. Mason jars work great for this!

For an interesting topping to fruit salads, do not strain the peaches from peach and honey vinegar. Mash them into the vinegar and drizzle over mixed fruits. Serve with warm toast which has been spread with honey cream.

Honey and cranberry vinegar is a colorful addition to any holiday menu. Make this unique condiment by cooking 3 cups cranberries in 1 cup apple cider vinegar. Simmer until the berries break open (at least 15 minutes). Add 1/2 cup clover honey and combine well. Store in a glass jar with a tight fitting lid and shake well before using on tossed salad greens. The cranberries add a welcome touch of brightness to winter salads.

Liquid Sweetener

Honey has special properties as a sweetener for hot liquids. It dissolves rapidly and brings a unique flavor to beverages. Honey is often used to sweeten teas and warm milk, but it is also an excellent way to enrich the taste of coffees and cold drinks.

Because, in equal amounts, honey is sweeter than sugar, be sure to use honey sparingly. One way to make it easier to use honey to sweeten liquids (hot or cold), is to dilute a cup of honey with 1/4 cup water. Store this thin liquid in a small pitcher. It will pour easily at any temperature.

You can also make frozen "honey cubes." Simply pour honey into an ice tray and allow to freeze. Empty these cubes into a ziplock bag and store in the freezer. These are a great way to add a quick touch of honey to a warm beverage while simultaneously bringing down the hot temperature. Mini ice cubes work better than full size, as you can regulate flavor more closely. These cubes are also a wonderful addition to a cool glass of ice tea during the warm summer months.

Prepare an easy breakfast chocolate by combining a spoonful each of cocoa and honey. Use a little boiling water to mix them well, then add a cup of warm milk.

For a cool honey-citrus chilled treat, combine a cup of lemon, orange, lime or grapefruit juice with about 1/4 cup honey. Add enough water to make a quart and serve over crushed ice. Make it even better by adding thinly sliced fruit.

A traditional hot weather cooler is made with honey-sweetened lemonade and ginger ale, topped with crushed fresh mint leaves.

The very best eggnog is always cooked with gentle care and then sweetened with one of the light, delicate honeys. Try a gentle clover honey for this one!

Drinks sweetened with honey have a long history of being both tasty and healthy. "mulse" is one of the oldest remedies based on honey.

Mulse is made by heating wine to the boiling point, then mixing in honey. In old-time England, mulse was often served at the beginning and end of meals.

The combination of hot wine and honey is an age-old restorative, credited with being able to hasten the healing of respiratory discomforts. It was also believed by many that a bit of honey-sweetened wine each day would ensure a long, vital life.

Some other ancient honey-sweetened drinks that were long thought to add to general health and well-being include:

• Old wine mixed with myrtle berries and honey

• Honey and any fresh fruit juice, especially the juice of mulberries

- Honey and water with an egg white beaten in

- Honey and milk

- Wine and honey with ginger, cinnamon, nutmeg or cloves

- Rose petals, honey and water

- Fermented grape juice and honey

- Unfermented grape juice and honey

- Wine, honey and pepper

When added to unfermented grape juice, honey was said to be a remedy for gout and nervous conditions.

Combined with wine and pepper, honey was used as a treatment for digestive ailments. This mixture was also said to be helpful for those affected with rheumatic disorders and maladies.

Hydromel

Water and honey, in the ancient world called "hydromel," was considered a medicine. It was used in many ways, some of which follow:

Serve hydromel to one recovering from serious illness and to invalids. It will give them strength and vigor.

Soothe a painful mouth by sipping on a light hydromel mixture.

A sore throat will cease to cause pain if warm hydromel is slowly sipped.

Ease discomfort of the stomach and belly by drinking regular doses of hydromel.

Hydromel will relieve a fever and encourage a swift recovery from illness.

Use generous amounts of hydromel to strengthen one with a weak constitution.

Regular use of hydromel made of spring water and local honey will sharpen the mind.

One who regularly partakes of hydromel will have a pleasant spirit, free from anger, sadness and infirmities of the mind.

Old English Mead

Mead is a mildly alcoholic liquid made from honey. Mead was, most likely, made long before wine or the cultivation of grapes.

Traditionally, liquid honey was gotten out of combs by opening the tops of the combs and then hanging them in a cloth bag. Liquid honey strained out into containers, leaving some of its sticky-sweet goodness on the cloth and in the broken combs.

The making of Old English mead began by soaking the empty combs and the cloth bags used for straining honey in water. Then this sweetened water was allowed to ferment.

Eventually, the making of mead became a highly competitive commercial undertaking. Each producer (like early vinegar producers) had a secret recipe that was fiercely guarded. And, as you can imagine, each producer's mead was slightly different than the next person's. This made for competition between the various producers.

Mead is honey and water that has been fermented by yeasts. The best mead is made to exacting standards. The beginning ratio of honey to water depends on the sugar content of the particular honey.

One way which was traditionally used to tell when water had enough honey melted into it to begin the fermentation process was to float an egg in the mixture. When the egg would all sink, except for a portion about the size of a small coin, the ratio was right.

The next step was to strain the liquid to remove impurities, such as pieces of comb. Then it was heated to the boiling point and put in a barrel to "work up." This could take a few days or even months.

Traditionally, the finest Old English mead was made of only honey and rain water. Fermenting agents, such as yeast, were provided by wild spores in the air.

Commercial makers soon found that the fermenting process could be hurried along by adding a starter, such as a piece of toast with yeast smeared on it.

If only part of the sugar content is converted by the yeast, sweet mead is produced. If all of the sugar is converted by the yeast, dry mead is produced.

Special commercial mead might be aged for years. Homemade kinds were often used immediately.

The exact recipe for a particular supplier's mead was considered a valuable secret, and always kept tightly guarded. The kind of honey, the source of the water, the kind of wood used in the barrels, the starter mix, the length of time for the aging process, were all things that influenced the final taste.

When the beginning mixture had a low sugar content, a light colored, dry or sparkling mead was made. When the beginning mixture had a high sugar content, a darker, sweet dessert mead was made.

Most 16th and 17th century English mead was pale gold in color and was said to sparkle like fine champagne.

The very first mead was, most likely, produced by an accident. Perhaps a bee's nest became flooded and the honey fermented naturally. Or, maybe some old honey in the bottom of a forgotten crock fermented.

In any case, man soon learned to turn honey into mead. Since early mead makers did not totally understand the action of yeasts on sugar, the process was considered something of a minor miracle. And so, it is not surprising that the mead itself was believed to have very special healing qualities.

In the Middle Ages, mead was often mixed with herbs to make healing tonics. Mead with herbs in it was called methiglin.

Methiglin was made by adding thyme, sweet marjoram, rosemary, ginger, cinnamon, bay leaves, cloves, pepper, sweetbriar leaves, mace, other spices or by adding fruits such as apples, pears, mulberries or quince to mead.

Folklore claims mead was able to impart on imbibers wisdom, immortality and the ability to write beautiful poetry.

Mead was said to protect the body from diseases of the brain. Mead was also prescribed for kidney ailments, gout and rheumatism. It served as a preventative as well as a curative.

England, however, was not the only country where mead was important.

Poland had a reputation as the home a very good mead. Monks at St. Basil made a mead flavored with hops. It was a famous remedy for treating both gout and rheumatism.

In addition to mead, honey is also used to make other forms of alcohol. And, it is often added to alcoholic drinks after fermentation to improve their flavor. Some honey drinks are:

- Cyser, made of fermented honey and apple juice, has a higher alcoholic content than cider.

- Scotland's famous Drambuie® is a combination of honey and whisky, in a secret combination.

- Athole brose, made of equal parts honey and cream, with Scotch whisky added to it, is considered a remedy for ills of many sorts.

- Krupnik is whisky boiled with honey and served while very hot.

Perhaps the most unique use of honey is found in an old Persian anecdote. It tells how to keep the master of the household in a sweet temper. A servant merely slips a straw into the sleeping master's mouth. Then a mixture of milk, honey and whisky is fed into it. This is supposed to ensure that the master's very first taste of the day is delicious.

Honey has more delicious uses than one might imagine. From mead and mulse to hydromel and on, the different ways honey has been closely intertwined into nearly every culture seems endless. And much of the love of honey comes from its unequaled taste in recipes from all over the world.

For a wonderful selection of honey recipes and concoctions, follow me along to the next chapter...

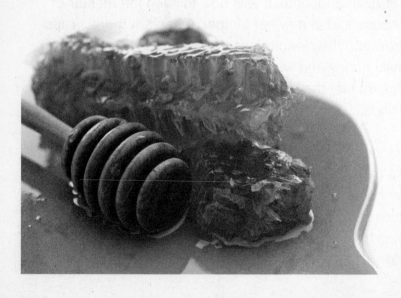

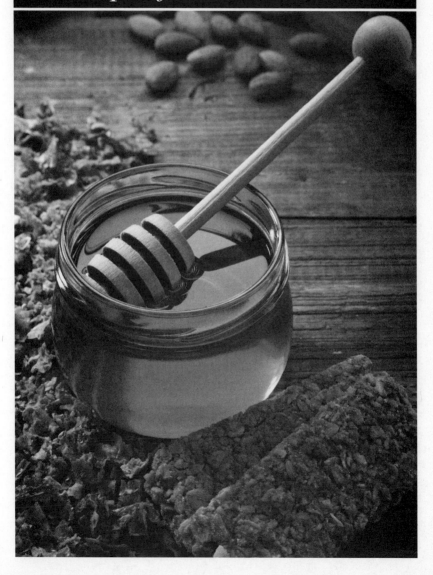

CHAPTER NINE

Recipes for Better Health

Cooking with honey can be a delicious way to add a natural sweetener, with the added benefit of vitamins and minerals, to your diet. It adds its unique flavor to liven up dressings and sauces, while making a sweet addition to breads and other baked goods. Honey has been used worldwide throughout history as a flavorful addition to everyday meals and dishes to gourmet entrees and confections.

Honey can also be used as a marvelous accompaniment to fresh buttermilk biscuits or on top of the morning's pancakes. It's delicious as a topping for ice cream or poured straight over fresh fruit.

This chapter will look at some fabulous ways to incorporate honey into your diet...deliciously!

But, before we get started, here are a few things to keep in mind when cooking with honey:

Heating honey
First, while many recipes call for honey to be cooked or heated, remember that high temperatures kill much of the nutritional value of honey, depleting it of its wonderful vitamins and minerals. It is okay to cook with honey, just keep an eye that the temperature does not get too hot.

When possible, honey should be added near the end of the cooking process in things like sauces. For baked goods recipes calling for honey, such as sweet breads, honey will need to be added at the beginning of the mixing process.

This will allow the sugar in the honey to act with the yeast to begin the rising action.

Some recipes suggest lowering the temperature of your oven by 25 degrees to offset some of the browning in baked goods caused by baking with honey.

Substituting Honey for Sugar
Honey is much sweeter than sugar, so when substituting it in your recipes, be aware of the difference and change measurements accordingly. As a rule of thumb, the amount of honey to be used in a recipe calling for sugar should be about two thirds to one half. In addition, honey contains more moisture than sugar, so you may wish to slightly reduce the amount of liquid in the original recipe to account for this. For recipes calling for more than a cup of sugar, substituting honey is not recommended, as the extra moisture honey brings tends to cause large changes in the consistency of baked goods.

Keep in mind that honey also has a different flavor than table sugar. It may affect, either positively or negatively, the flavor outcome of your baked goods.

You may wish to add 1/4 teaspoon baking soda to the batter of baked goods that have had honey substituted for cane sugar. This will help offset some of honey's acidic taste in the final product.

When substituting honey for cane sugar, you may notice one or all of these traits in your final product. Knowing what the differences are ahead of time will allow you to make adjustments to the recipe:

- Honey has more moisture content than sugar

- Honey is more dense than sugar, and will give you a weightier baked good

- Honey browns faster than recipes made with sugar

- Honey is nearly twice as sweet as sugar, thus needing less in the recipe

- Honey is slightly higher in calories, although you will not need to use as much

- Honey adds acid to the recipe

- Honey tends to brown baked goods, such as cakes and cookies, at a faster rate than sugar

- Honey adds its own, unique flavor to recipes, and if too pungent a honey is used, it will certainly alter the flavor of the final product

- Honey brings more vitamins and minerals to a recipe than its counterpart in sugar

- Honey, because of its preservation qualities, can lengthen the freshness time in baked goods

Weights and Measures

One cup of honey equals roughly 12 ounces on the scale.

In most recipes, you can substitute 3/4 to 1/2 cup of honey in the place of one full cup of cane sugar.

Honey Tip

When using honey and vegetable oil in the same recipe, measure out the vegetable oil in your measuring cup first. Then measure the honey. Using vegetable oil first will coat the measuring cup and allow the honey to slide out easier.

Now Let's Get Cooking!

Honey Pepper Rub

This sweet and savory rub is perfect for steaks on the grill.

1/4 cup honey
6 cloves garlic, minced
2 t kosher salt
2 t paprika
2 t dry mustard
2 t fresh ground black pepper
Dash onion salt

Combine all the ingredients together in a small bowl. Use as a rub on steaks. Rub can be placed on meat and allowed to rest for at least 15 minutes prior to grilling.

Taylor's Honey Cake

This recipe is so moist and delicious it can even be served alone, without frosting, for those watching extra calories!

2 c. flour	1/4 c water
1 c. sugar	1 T baking powder
1/2 c. honey	2 t. vanilla extract
1 c. vegetable oil	3 eggs

1. Combine dry ingredients in a mixing bowl, making a well in center of ingredients.

2. In a medium bowl, combine vegetable oil, honey and water.

3. Add wet ingredients to the bowl of dry ingredients and beat with an electric mixer until combined.

4. Add vanilla extract and eggs and continue beating on medium speed for two minutes.

5. Pour into a greased and floured 9"x13" baking dish and bake in a preheated oven at 350° for 25-40 minutes. Cake is done when the center springs back after gently being touched.

6. Serve warm, or cool completely and frost with honey frosting.

Honey Lollipops

These honey lollipops are an excellent way to soothe a sore, irritated throat or help bring relief to a nagging cough.

1/3 cup honey	1 T water
1 cup sugar	Candy sticks
3 T light corn syrup	

1. Line a cookie sheet or tray with wax paper.

2. In a heavy pan, add honey, sugar, corn syrup and water. Cook over medium heat until mixture is dissolved and combined.

3. Continue cooking until mixture has reached 300°F when checked with a candy thermometer.

4. Pour small dollops of candy solution onto wax paper (or use a candy mold). Quickly add candy sticks making sure honey solution encompasses the sticks.

5. Allow to cool completely, about 20 minutes.

6. Gently peel back wax paper from lollipops. Wrap in plastic or additional wax paper and store in a cool, dry place until ready to use.

For a special treat, feel free to add your favorite flavoring to these honey pops as well. Flavoring oils such as lemon, cinnamon or even anise work especially well, but any flavoring will work!

Honey Glazed Ham

1-10 pound fully cooked ham
1/2 cup honey
1/2 cup molasses
1/2 cup light brown or muscovado sugar
2 T dijon mustard
1/4 cup pineapple juice
Cloves

1. Combine honey, molasses, brown or muscovado sugar, mustard and pineapple juice in a heavy bottom pan until well incorporated. Cook over medium heat until boiling; let simmer 5-10 minutes longer until juices begin to thicken. Remove from heat.

2. Place ham in a foil-lined roasting pan. Make long cuts into the ham in a diamond shape about an inch apart. Place cloves into the center of each diamond (this part is optional).

3. Carefully brush or spoon glaze over ham. Cover with aluminum foil to allow ham to self-baste in its' juices. If necessary, add water to pan (not over ham) to allow to keep moist.

4. Bake at 350° for two hours. Baste ham again and continue to re-baste every 30 minutes until ham has reached desired temperature when checked with a meat thermometer.

Honey Applesauce

Instead of making your own honey from scratch, you can eliminate the apples from this recipe and continue to directions to sweeten up jars of store bought applesauce.

12-15 medium apples
2 cups apple juice
Water as needed
1/2 cup honey
3-4 t cinnamon

1. Core, peel and cut apples into chunks. Place in a large cooking pot with a heavy bottom over medium-high heat. Add apple juice.

2. Cook apples for about 30-40 minutes, until they are mushy. Add water as needed to keep juicy, but not too watery.

3. For thinner applesauce, add more water. For a thicker applesauce, allow some of the juices to cook off over simmering heat.

4. Take off burner and allow to cool a bit. Add 1/2 cup of honey and cinnamon to taste.

5. Can serve warm or refrigerate for later use.

Honey Baked Apples

Honey-baked apples are a traditional food throughout European countries.

4 apples
pinch nutmeg
pinch cinnamon
honey

1. Wash and remove the cores from well-ripened apples. Granny Smith, Fuji and Melrose work well.

2. Arrange apples in a baking dish and drizzle a tablespoon or two of honey over each apple.

3. Sprinkle with nutmeg and cinnamon and bake at 350° until the apples are well done and tender.

Honey Fruit Dip

Try this wonderful tip served cool with an assortment of fresh strawberries, grapes, cantaloupe and honeydew.

4 oz whipped cream cheese
3 T marshmallow cream
1 T honey

Combine all ingredients together until well mixed. Serve cold.

Honey Sauce

This is a great sauce to be served on the side along with vegetables, like broccoli or peas. Also delicious over a cooked vegetable medley or chef's salad.

Also, there is no need to add salt to this recipe, as the celery has a natural salting effect. Great for people who are watching their salt intake!

3 stalks celery
1/3 cup balsamic vinegar
3 Tablespoons honey

1. Combine all ingredients in a blender until smooth.

2. Can be served at room temperature or slightly warmed.

Honey Fruit Glaze

This glaze is good for topping breads, or favorite cuts of meat such as pork, chicken or beef.

1/2 cup honey
1/4 cup fruit juice (orange, lemon, pineapple or apricot)
finely chopped fruit

1. Combine honey and fruit juice in a blender.

2. Add a few tablespoons of finely chopped fruit and combine. Top on favorite cut of meat.

Honey Frosting

Honey frosting is an quick topping for baked goods.

4 oz honey
8 oz cream cheese, softened
lemon juice

1. Beat cream cheese in a mixing bowl until fluffy.
2. Add honey and a splash of lemon juice and incorporate completely. Continue beating for 1 minute
3. Spread on a cooled cake.

Sprinkle slivered almonds on top or ground walnuts for a special touch.

Whipped Honey Frosting

Try this whipped honey frosting made with egg whites.

1 cup honey
2 egg whites
lemon juice

1. Pour honey into a saucepan and boil until it reaches the soft ball stage (238°-240°).

2. Beat eggs whites until they reach stiff consistency

3. Pour warmed honey over the stiffly beaten egg whites and beat until the frosting is spreadable consistency.

Honey Cookies

The oldest (and easiest to make) honey cookies are merely a concoction of warm honey and flour.

1/2 cup honey
1-1/2 cup flour

1. Stir honey and flour together. Once combined, knead into a soft dough.

2. Roll dough out onto a sheet of wax paper, keeping them about a half an inch thick.

3. Cover dough and let set overnight in the refrigerator.

4. Cut into squares or use cookie cutters to shape.

5. Bake at 300° until cookies are very lightly browned. Seal cookies in airtight container.

Honey Cream

Honey cream is another especially good, and good-for-you, bread topping

1/4 cup honey
1/4 cup + 2T heavy cream

Heat honey until it is warm, but not hot. Mix in honey and combine well. Store in refrigerator.

Honey Butter I

Use this delicious topping on toast and fresh bread.

1/4 cup honey
1/4 cup butter
orange zest (optional)

1. Combine honey and butter together.
2. Store in the refrigerator in a butter crock, or form into a ball.

Add a bit of grated orange peel for extra goodness.

Honey Butter II

1 cup butter, softened (2 sticks); do not use margarine
1/2 c honey
1/2 t vanilla extract

1. Place butter sticks in mixing bowl and beat until creamy. Add honey and vanilla and resume beating until whipped and well blended.

2. Scoop honey butter into a small butter crock or wrap in wax paper and form into a log roll. Cool in refrigerator until firmed up a bit.

3. Store in refrigerator.

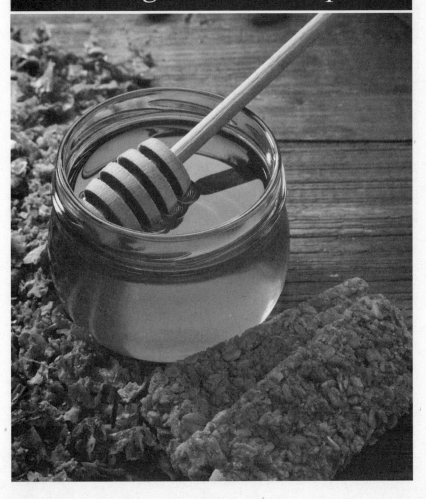

CHAPTER TEN
Just for Fun:
Bees & Honey
In Legend & Worship

Mankind's love affair with honey goes back thousands of years. Paintings etched on rock cliffs near Valencia, Spain show one of the ways our early ancestors gathered honey. Some of our oldest histories indicate honey taking was being perfected among the lake dwellers of Switzerland.

Much of what ancient peoples knew about honey was shrouded in both myth and legend. Even as recently as the days of the Roman Empire the Roman scholar, Pliny, speculated honey must be either sweat from the sky or spit from stars. And, it has been used as a symbol of everlasting bliss, as Egyptian kings expected to be amply supplied with lotus blossoms, honey and honey cakes, even in death.

Over the ages, from witchcraft and myth to reverence and worship, honey has been praised as being something pure in an otherwise impure world. Honey's seemingly miraculous sweetness, combined with its surprising power to heal, has provided comfort for and wonder for uncounted generations.

The Royal Bee
Centuries rich in history have long depicted the bee as metaphorically symbolic of kings or nobility.

For example in Egypt of long ago, the bee was the hieroglyphic which was symbolic for a king. The bee symbol was used this way gracing cavern walls and early historical writings for nearly 4000 years.

Kings in ancient India were anointed with honey before their coronations.

In France, the Bonapartes used bees as their emblem. Napoleon Bonaparte, Emperor of France, had bees stitched onto his royal cape, perhaps by Josephine his wife, and his green coronation robes were covered with golden bees as symbols of both his reign of power and intended immortality.

Honey in Ritual and Legend

Biblically, both Egypt and Canaan are referred to as lands which flow with milk and honey. In Biblical types, milk and honey were both symbols of great wealth and abundance.

In most all cultures all throughout the world honey has been considered the elixir of love. In the epitome of love laced folklore, Cupid is said to have dipped his arrows of love in fresh honey before launching them to their intended targets.

Rituals

Honey has a long history of use in rituals surrounding important events, such as birth, marriage and death. The practice of giving babies a dab of honey at birth dates back to prehistoric times. (This was long before honey was found to have what we now know as botulism and potentially dangerous for infant consumption.) Often honey was offered even before the baby's first taste of mother's milk.

Poetry, from nations all across the world, compares the sweetness of love to that of honey. It is the traditional remedy for a broken heart. Honey has also been considered a magical elixir of love with aphrodisiac properties. For that reason, honey is still featured in the marriage ceremonies of many cultures even today.

Even the first, sweetest month of marriage has its honey connection. The term "honeymoon" probably originated because the first month of marriage is considered to be the sweetest.

Many folktales in various cultures believe that if you smear honey on the lintel and door posts of a new home those who live there will have their lives filled with goodness and sweetness.

Traditionally, guests at Hindu wedding feasts were served honey. Then the bride's forehead, lips, eyelids and ear lobes would be anointed with honey, to keep her sweet. Also, the honey's purity was thought able to repel any evil spirits that happened to show up during the marriage celebration. Because of the honey's protection, the newlyweds could expect years of happiness.

And, in India, the groom was expected to dine on honey on his wedding day. This was to ensure the couple's fertility.

Croatian grooms also had their homes' thresholds smeared with honey before the bride came across it.

Both bride and groom in a Balkan wedding had their faces smeared with honey. This made sure they would find each other nice and sweet.

In early Rome, the traditional wedding banquet included a drink made of honey, milk and poppy juice. Supposedly, this special liquid made those who drank it dizzy and happy. It also was reported to bring about sweet dreams.

In Roman times, taxes were often paid in honey. Because of the reputation of the honey in the Pontus area, those living there had to pay their taxes in wax instead of honey.

In olden Germany, a baby's lips were often smeared with honey at birth. This early feeding "proved" it had a soul, and so protected it from the father's right to have the newborn killed if it was not wanted.

In India, honey was considered the best first nourishment for babies. Babies of Greeks, Germans and Hebrews were fed honey immediately after birth, too.

Greek culture considered honey an elixir of perpetual youth. It was also considered capable of conveying the ability to make sweet, pleasant words. Plato, Sophocles, Xenophon, Virgil, St. Ambrose, and St. Basil were considered to be wise and eloquent because each one had bees land on their mouths when they were babies.

It is widely believed that the builders of the fabulous city of Babylon began by sprinkling its foundation with honey, oil and wine.

Both Sumerian and Babylonian priests used honey in rites for exorcizing evil spirits and demons.

In some cultures, honey was poured on the hands of new priests to make them spiritually clean and undefiled. Other purification ceremonies mix honey with butter and milk curds. This was used by old-time priests and priestesses to exorcise evil spirits, consecrate temples, and as food for new initiates. Both honey and milk products were widely used as symbols of riches and plenty.

Embalming

Liquid which seeped from the embalmed dead was believed by the ancients to have great medicinal qualities.

Immersing a body in honey was one of the earliest ways of preserving the dead. It proved to be a very good preservative for a corpse, and may have once been the only process available to people. Using this method of honey immersion to preserve dead bodies was common among the Babylonian peoples. The Babylonians and Assyrians also preserved bodies by covering them with beeswax, then putting them in honey to retard decay.

History is rich with stories of kings and warriors being forever entombed in honey:

- Homer's Odyssey indicates that Achilles, after taking that deadly arrow in his heel, was buried in honey.

- At his death Alexander the Great, by his own order, was placed in white honey in a golden coffin.

- Herod I, King of Judaea, had his beautiful wife, Marianne, executed. Then he kept her body near him for seven years – all the while preserved in honey.

- The Greek historian, Herodotus, wrote that the Scythians enclosed bodies of dead kings in beeswax.

It was long believed there was great healing power in a mummy. One ancient recipe begins with embalming directions for making the mummy:

Take one man-child and raise him up well-fed on fruits. When his is about 30 years old, put him into a crock hewn of a single stone and sprinkle him with herbs and spices. Then fill the crock to the very top with honey and seal it tight for at least 100 years.

In Burma, honey was once considered such pure, incorruptible stuff that it could be reused -- and sold in the marketplace -- even after it had been used for preservation of a dead body!

Magic Wax
Sorcerers once used beeswax for making likenesses of both people and animals. Then, if the waxen figure was damaged or destroyed it was believed that the one it represented would suffer or die, too.

Beeswax models were used by the magicians of Egypt, Babylonia and India. Wizards and witches used them in Europe, too.

In Babylonia and Assyria it was believed that if an unfriendly wizard put a waxen image of a man near a corpse, great evil would surely come to that man.

The Romans often used beeswax to make images of people they disliked. They felt they could cause these people misfortune and physical harm, much like the implications of modern day voodoo dolls.

One old, old story is told of a man who made a beeswax model of a crocodile, then put in into the pool where his wife's lover bathed. The wax crocodile turned into a live crocodile, and soon solved the man's problems. Its job done, the crocodile then turned back into a waxen image.

Beeswax was not always used for evil purposes. It also was used to 'heal' wounded pottery.

You probably know that the word "sincere" can mean genuine, honest, and true. All these words refer to the use of beeswax, because our word "sincere" was formed from the Latin "sin" for without and "cere" for wax.

Literally, sincere originally translates into the phrase "without wax." This is because when pottery was fired in the kiln, cracks would sometimes develop. These imperfections could be "healed" by filling them with beeswax and then re-firing the piece. And so, the more valuable, perfect-the-first-time pottery was created without wax, and so was "sincere" pottery.

The Power of Bees

Because honey is such a wondrous substance, it is no surprise that the bees which produce it came to have a very special place in many cultures. Beekeeping was a respected pursuit, undertaken by monks and scholars, as well as farmers.

The Greek philosopher and teacher, Aristotle, was a serious beekeeper. He studied the ways of the bees as part of his quest to understand the workings of the universe.

Fortunately for him, Virgil, the famous Roman poet, was also a keeper of bees. When a band of soldiers came to raid his home his servants hid the household valuables among his beehives. When the soldiers approached, Virgil's bees attacked them and saved their master's possessions.

Folklore in several countries describe a very ancient and saintly bee that was white (or very light in color).

In East Africa, a clan with a bee totem, claims to have the power to make bees follow them.

Many people believe a person can whistle or make other noise to attract bees.

In Europe, the practice of talking to bees as members of the family is widespread. Bees are treated as important members of the family. Whenever any significant event occurs, the family bees must be formally told about it.

Family arguments are not permitted in front of the family's bees, or near their hives. If the beekeeper dies, someone must go to the hives and explain to the bees what happened, so that they, too, do not die.

As part of many weddings in Bavaria and Bohemia the family bee hives are decorated with red cloth when there is a wedding in household. This way, the bees can share in the family's happiness.

Russian families place a cup of honey by the casket at a funeral. This is the bee's final gift to the loved one's departed.

Folklore in both Scotland and Germany tells of how souls, in the form of bees, come out of people's bodies while they sleep.

In many places, no one will buy the bees of a dead man. It is thought to be a bad investment, because the bees are likely to fly away to look for their dead master.

Africa and India both have traditions of believing bees can tell the future.

In China, a day on which the family's bees swarm is considered to be a lucky day for members of the household.

Bees are said to have foreknowledge of the weather. If the bees go out, it is safe for the family to do so. If the bees stay in their hive, it is considered dangerous for the family to go out, too.

Many people in southern Europe feel it is not good to feed honey to one who is seriously ill. This is not because it will harm the person, but because if the person eats the honey and then dies, the bees will be so upset they, too, will die.

Legendary Home Remedies
Home remedies using honey throughout the ages are legendary.

Assyria's ancient "Book of Medicines" used honey in over 300 prescriptions, and beeswax in more than 50! It was long believed that honey's healing properties was the cornerstone in many important remedies.

In Asia, honey was traditionally used to affect the fertility of women, cattle and crops.

Early Mediterranean peoples believed honey prevented blight and pestilence from attacking their lands.

Perhaps the greatest physicist who ever lived, Democritus, was a devoted honey enthusiast. After living for more than 100 years, he decided he had lived long enough and stopped eating, to hasten his end. When told that his immediate death would be an inconvenience, because of an upcoming holiday, he agreed to have some honey so he would live until it was more convenient for those around him to have a funeral.

In second and third century China, honey and opium were mixed together for special remedies.

It has been said that honey gathered just after seeing a rainbow has special power to cure disease.

Homer is reputed to have prospered on a diet of honey, barley flour, wine and cheese made from goat's milk.

Roman soldiers carried honey in their gear to use for treating wounds.

Hippocrates, considered the father of modern medicine, prescribed a daily dose of honey for those who wished to live a long life. He also gave a recipe for a honey-based aphrodisiac. It was made of ass's meat, milk and honey.

In Istanbul, honey was regularly given to members of the local harems to promote good spirits.

The Greeks author, Theophrastus, said honey would keep hair from falling off the head. Many other Greek remedies used honey as part of healing salves.

A popular old time cure-all for gray hair began with gathering a fresh handful of bees. Then, one cooked them in oil and rubbed them into the hair. It was guaranteed to turn gray hair black.

Both the Greeks and the Romans used fresh honey as a laxative.

The Romans called honey, with or without milk, the very best sleeping potion.

Greeks athletes were traditionally given honey after competing in their Olympic games. It was said to banish fatigue and revitalize the athletes.

Sweet Dreams
It is said that if you dream of honey you will soon resolve a problem.

If you dream about honey, your personal life will be sweet and fulfilling.

Dream about a beehive and you will soon find that riches will come your way.

If you dream about a beehive that is angry and disturbed, you have done something to bring you trouble and heartache.

Should you suffer a bee sting in a dream, expect good luck to come your way.

Dream of dead bees and expect something bad to happen to a close friend.

Hear the buzzing of bees in a dream and you will soon receive good news.

If you dream of eating honey while it is still in the comb you can expect to be rewarded with happiness and wealth.

Bees & Honey in Worship

Honey has, since time began, been part of holy writings. To the early Hebrews the idea of a wonderful land of their own was one which offered an abundance of "milk and honey." Twenty-one times in the Old Testament of the Bible the "Promised Land" is described as "flowing with milk and honey. In all, 56 Bible verses mention honey.

Often, it was sent as gift to those from whom one was seeking favor. For example, Jacob sent honey to the governor of Egypt and Jeroboam sent honey to a prophet when he asked for healing for his son.

Early Christians presented newly baptized persons with a mixture of milk and honey.

Milk and honey were used as part of the Eucharist in the Catholic Church until about the year 600.

Telling of riddles was once a common pastime. Samson's honey riddle is one of the oldest known riddles. "Out of the eater came something to eat, and out of the strong came something sweet."

Deborah was one of the many judges of the Old Testament. Her name means "bee," possibly because they were considered wise creatures.

The only thing in the Bible that was sweeter than honey was manna, which was considered six times sweeter than honey.

Clement of Alexandria, the Greek theologian and religious writer, compared milk and honey. He wrote that milk was like the nourishment needed after earthly birth and honey was like the food needed after spiritual birth.

The patron saint of beekeepers is St. Ambrose. When he was a baby a swarm of bees is said to have settled on his mouth. In Spain, St. John of the Nettles is said to be the patron saint of bees. Women go to his tomb to pray that the child they are carrying will be a boy. In the Ukraine, the patron saint of beekeepers is St. Sossima.

One ancient tradition says that the very first swarm of bees was the one that flew out of Paradise in sadness at the fall of man.

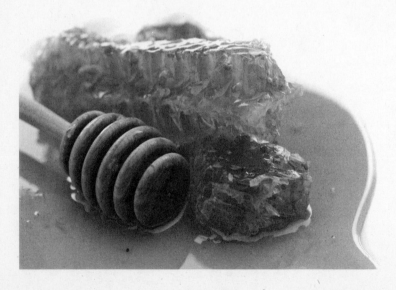

168

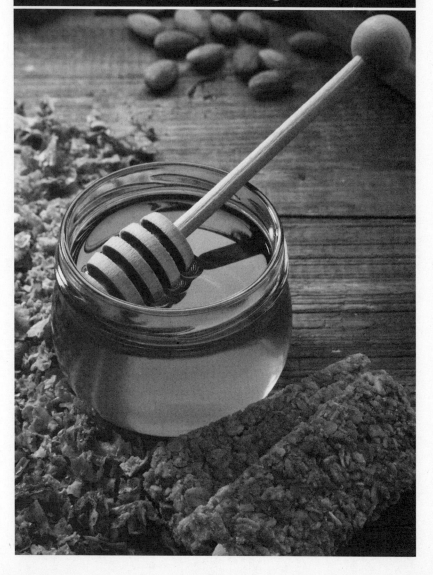

CHAPTER ELEVEN
Frequently Asked Questions

How long does honey last?

When stored correctly, honey (like sugar) lasts indefinitely and does not go bad.

What is the proper way to store honey? Does it need to be refrigerated?

Honey should be stored in an airtight jar or container out of the path of direct sunlight.

Remember when storing honey, that honey absorbs moisture and odors. Do not store honey with anything likely to spread odor to the honey and ruin its delicate flavor and aroma.

Honey does not need to be refrigerated, although it can be refrigerated without ruining the honey. Honey that has been stored in the refrigerator sometimes develops "crystals." These crystals are completely harmless and do not affect honey's aroma or flavor, only its texture. Crystallization in the honey does not mean it has gone bad.

Why has my honey become cloudy? Is cloudy honey still safe to eat?

Honey that has become cloudy has merely begun the crystallization process. Tiny sugar crystals have started to form. Honey that has become cloudy is perfectly safe to eat.

If you prefer, the honey can be restored back to its clear state with gentle heating.

How can I reconstitute honey that has been crystallized?

Honey that has begun to crystallize is perfectly safe for consumption. However, if you prefer, honey can be reconstituted back into its full, original liquid state.

Changing honey crystals back to a liquid can be done several ways.

Place the honey in a saucepan and slowly and gently raise the temperature, stirring often, until the honey crystals have reconstituted. Be sure not to heat the honey to a high temperature, as this will destroy much of its nutritional and remedial value.

Or, you can place the jar of honey (with the lid on) in a bowl of warm water until the crystals have dissolved back into the honey.

Microwaving can also be used. But, since the temperature of microwaves are more difficult to regulate, this method may produce too much heat for the honey to remain in its most raw form. Proceed with caution.

Which honey is best for using as a home remedy aid?

Raw honey is the purest form of honey and contains the most properties for home remedies and treatments. It has undergone little or no heat pasteurization which can destroy most of honey's most beneficial elements.

What is raw honey?

Raw honey is considered the most pure form of honey, straight from the beehive. Raw honey has not undergone the heated pasteurization process, thus it has kept its nutritional value intact. Raw honey also contains "propolis" or "bee glue" that is very beneficial in home health remedies. Pollen spores from local plants are also present in raw honey, making it a preferred treatment for some sufferers of allergies.

It is in this state that honey presents the most antibacterial, antifungal and antiviral properties.

Where can I purchase raw honey?

Raw honey can be purchased at a variety of places. Try checking out reputable bee farmers, Amish farms, local farmers markets, State fairs, gourmet food shops, health food shops, organic food retailers and of course online.

To ensure you are getting the most benefit from your raw honey, try to purchase honey from local farmers and bee keepers.

Why should I purchase honey from local sources?

Honey taken from local hives (within a few miles from your home) tend to have the same pollen spores you are accustomed to around your own home. Many home remedies state that eating honey taken from local hives helps to desensitize your body's system against these types of allergies.

Is honey harmful to babies?

It could be. Honey may contain Clostridium bacteria which could cause botulism poisoning.

Honey should never be given to an infant under one year of age. After one year of age, children's immune systems strengthen and are better able to combat bacteria.

What are the different grades of honey?

The USDA has established a voluntary grading system for honey.

In short, honey rated grade A is considered quality honey. It is listed as "good" honey, containing very few, if any, artifacts or particles. It contains the least amount of water of the honey grades (less than 18%) and has good flavor and aroma. It's consistency is clear, other than the possibility of a few tiny bubbles left from the packaging process. Grade A honey may contain pollen spores. This is perfectly fine, and can, in fact, be beneficial.

Grade B honey is considered "reasonably good" honey. It may contain slightly more artifacts than grade A honey, although still few in number. Grade B honey contains the same water content as grade A honey, with a reasonably good flavor and aroma.

Grade C honey is considered "fairly good" on the honey scale. It contains more artifacts than grades A or B, although still not enough to alter edibility or appearance.

Grade C honey has a slightly higher water content (less than 20% water), and fairly clear appearance with some particles.

There is also a substandard grade of honey. This honey may have too many particles or changes in appearance or flavor to warrant a higher grade.

I purchased a jar of honey, but the label does not indicate what grade it is. How can I tell whether my honey is of good quality or not?

There are several ways one can test honey for its quality.

Honey should always be clear and consistent in its color. There should never be a layering of color within honey, or sediment on the bottom of the honey jar. If the honey is golden, it should be golden throughout. If the honey is dark, it should maintain its darker color throughout the bottle.

When pouring honey, the highest quality honey should flow evenly and without clumping or breaking off. Many people recommend taking a butter knife or spoon and dipping it into a jar of honey. Raise the utensil and let the honey fall back off into the bottle. It should glide off smoothly without uneven clumping or breakage and should not drip off in large drops.

Can honey be substituted for sugar?

Honey can be an acceptable substitution for sugar in many recipes.

Honey is naturally sweeter than sugar, so one needs to be careful to adjust the recipe accordingly. For baked goods, 1/2 to 3/4 cup of honey can be substituted in place of 1 cup of sugar.

Honey also tends to bake darker quicker. You may wish to adjust your oven's temperature by turning it down 25° to prevent darkening.

In addition, honey contains more liquid than cane sugar. Try lessening the recipe's liquid content by a tablespoon or two to make up for this.

Honey does contain slightly more calories than sugar, but offsets this by the fact that you need less honey for sweetening.

Remember that honey comes in all different flavors and aromas. Adding one of these in the place of sugar can bring an entirely new taste to the dish. Enjoy experimenting!

Is bee pollen in honey safe to eat?

Not only do researchers say pollen in honey is safe to eat, many believe the pollen can help immunize against allergies. Bee pollen also is known to contain numerous vitamins, minerals and enzymes that are beneficial to the human body.

I have recently seen bottles of sugar-free honey in stores. Is this really honey?

No. There is no such things as true, sugar-free honey. Honey which is labeled as sugar-free is not honey at all, but a look-alike product that uses a honey flavoring to achieve its taste.

Is it okay to chew on raw honeycomb?
Yes, chewing on raw honeycomb is perfectly safe. In fact, it is a wonderful source of unprocessed, raw honey. It contains the most vitamins and minerals, and you can be certain it has not undergone pasteurization which destroys so much of honey's health benefits.

Is honey a good alternative for diabetic patients?
Many diabetics use honey, in moderation, as an alternative to cane sugar and artificial sweeteners. One benefit of honey, is that unlike sugar, its release into the digestive system is more prolonged. This slower absorption allows blood sugar levels to be raised gradually, without spiking which is common after consuming many sugary foods.

But honey is still a substance which can raise blood sugar levels. And, everyone's body is different in the way that it reacts to outside stimuli. Always be sure and consult your physician if you have questions about your diabetes and whether a moderate intake in honey is advisable for diabetic patients.

What is Royal Jelly?

Royal Jelly is the name of the food nurse bees produce. It is excreted from the pharyngeal glands in their heads after they have eaten lots of pollen.

Royal jelly is rich in both proteins and vitamins. It can be found as an active ingredient in many of today's skin care products, or sold independently and used as a skin moisturizer.

Historically, royal jelly was considered something used by royalty and was not commonly available to others.

What is Bee's Wax?

In the hive, bees wax is the foundational element for honeycombs. It general takes about 10 pounds of honey to produce a single pound of bees wax.

Bees wax has countless uses in everything from moustache wax and furniture polish to a preserving cheese coating and candle formation.

What is Propolis?

Propolis is a resinous substance that can be found around leaf buds and on the bark of trees. Honeybees gather it to patch holes in the hive and to use as a protective film around anything that dies in the hive.

Some research studies are showing promising results for the use of propolis as a healing agent.

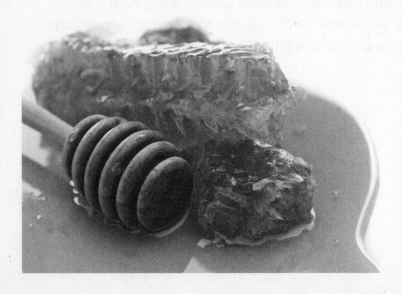

Additional books by Emily Thacker

Additional books by Emily Thacker
can be ordered using the attached order form
at the back of this book,
or by visiting our website at
http://www.jamesdirect.com

THE VINEGAR BOOK

Everyone loves vinegar! Its piquant bite blends well with an endless number of other foods. It tenderizes, enhances and preserves foods. More importantly, vinegar is a terrific germ killer. It is active against bacteria, viruses, molds and fungus. This safe, healing food can be found all across the world in many forms and flavors.

It is the traveler's friend, as it helps to prevent the system upsets that often plague tourists. Research has shown it to be effective in killing flu germs. It is also known for its anti-itch properties and its muscle soothing abilities.

Vinegar's long history as a panacea for the aches and pains of this world is respected in many cultures and places. Anyone who is serious about natural healing, old time remedies or folk medicine *must* have this book! (Also consider *THE VINEGAR ANNIVERSARY BOOK,* a blending of four separate books on vinegar: *THE VINEGAR BOOK, THE VINEGAR BOOK II, THE VINEGAR HOME GUIDE and THE VINEGAR DIET.)*

To find out more about *THE VINEGAR BOOK*, see the publisher's website: http://www.jamesdirect.com or buy it using the order form at the end of this book.

Excerpts from
THE VINEGAR BOOK

"Make your own instant window cleaner cloth! Combine 1/2 teaspoon liquid soap, 1/4 cup vinegar, and 2 cups water. Soak a sponge or small cloth in this mixture, then wring it out. Store the window cleaner cloth in a glass jar with a tight fitting lid until needed. Then simply wipe spots and smears from dirty windows. They will clean up without streaks – no mess, no fuss."

"Heat 1 cup herbal vinegar to the boiling point and pour it into a large bowl. Lean over the bowl and drape a towel over your head and the bowl. Allow the warm, moist steam to soften facial skin. When the vinegar has cooled, pat it onto the face as a cleansing astringent. Strawberry vinegar is especially good for the skin."

"Research in Japan is beginning to reveal the way vinegar works to sustain good health and slow down aging. It is believed that vinegar can help the body by interfering with the formation of fatty peroxides. This affects good health and long life in two very important ways..."

"To prevent anemia, the body needs iron, B-12, folate and a wide range of other nutrients. Apple cider vinegar delivers many of these nutrients, in an easy to digest and absorbable form."

"The time-honored vinegar recipe for dealing with arthritis is 1 teaspoon honey and 1 teaspoon apple cider vinegar, mixed into a glass of water and taken morning and evening.

GARLIC:
NATURE'S NATURAL COMPANION

This volume is a celebration of the miraculous healing powers of garlic! Across the world, it is used as a vegetable, a health food and to empower the immune system. Garlic has an almost endless number of aromatic compounds that constantly react with air and the foods it comes into contact with. These complex new mixtures produce the tantalizing aromas associated with this remarkable vegetable.

From earliest times garlic's ability to kill germs and heal sickness has been recognized. It has been used as an amulet to frighten away vampires and combined with vinegar to make the Thieves' Vinegar that reputedly offered protection from the plague.

Garlic grows almost everywhere, from the cold of Siberia and Tibet to the warmth of the Mediterranean and sunny California. Much of the world's supply is grown in China, who ships it out by the ton. It comes in tiny, intense, almost bitter bulbs to large elephant garlic bulbs.

The wonder of this versatile food is celebrated in festivals and fairs. Cook offs feature it in surprising recopies. Garlic is truly one of the healthiest, most widely used healing foods on the planet!

To find out more about *GARLIC: NATURE'S NATURAL COMPANION*, see the publisher's website: http://www.jamesdirect.com or buy it using the order form at the end of this book.

Excerpts from
GARLIC:
NATURE'S NATURAL COMPANION

"Garlic is listed as number one on the National Cancer Institute's list of foods which are potential cancer preventatives. Herbert Pierson, director of the Institute's study, says garlic has the most potential of all foods as a cancer fighting substance. Because of this the National Cancer Institute is sponsoring a five year, multi-million dollar study. They hope to determine exactly what garlic does in the body, how it does it, and how much garlic is needed to do the job."

"A bowl of chicken soup with lots of garlic in it will help to drive away a cold."

"Many scientists believe substances in this fortified vinegar deter the spread of prostate cancers. The chemicals that are so abundant in this mix of foods have actually killed some kinds of cancer."

"Add a mild garlic flavor to mashed potatoes by simply boiling whole garlic cloves along with the potatoes. For a stronger taste of garlic, mash the garlic into the potatoes. Or, you can simply add roasted or boiled garlic as you mash the potatoes."

"If you drink a cup of garlic tea every day, you will keep high blood pressure from developing."

THE MAGIC OF BAKING SODA

Do you keep your baking soda in the refrigerator or in the medicine cabinet? Or, perhaps you keep it with your laundry or cleaning supplies? Whether you call it bicarbonate of soda, sodium bicarbonate, bread soda ... or plain old baking soda ... this remarkable powder has hundreds of uses. You will want to keep it in your kitchen, medicine cabinet and with your cleaning and laundry supplies.

Baking soda is a naturally occurring substance that is kind to the environment. It is used to soothe allergies, exactly the opposite of many harsh chemical cleaning supplies. Most of the world's baking soda comes from a single huge deposit located in Wyoming.

Whether it is to soothe an acid stomach or the itching of rashes, baking soda is a must-have for the medicine cabinet. It is used in hospitals to protect the kidneys from intravenous dyes used in CT scans and to assist in dialysis treatments. Make sure you are getting all the benefits possible from this inexpensive substance you already have in your home.

To find out more about *THE MAGIC OF BAKING SODA*, see the publisher's website: http://www.jamesdirect.com or buy it using the order form at the end of this book.

Excerpts from
THE MAGIC OF BAKING SODA

"The prestigious Journal of the American Society of Nephrology reports that patients with chronic kidney disease can slow the progression of their renal failure by taking daily supplements of baking soda. This, doctors have found, works because a common complication of chronic kidney disease is a condition called metabolic acidosis. This shortage of plasma bicarbonate can be relieved by taking baking soda on a daily basis."

"When about a third of a cup of baking soda is added to a washer load of clothes, the amount of bleach needed to remove stains is cut in half."

"Plastic deck furniture and vinyl chairs can look beautiful again after being cleaned with a baking soda paste. This is a great deck furniture cleaner for both beginning and end-of-season clean up."

"Sprinkle baking soda on the soil around your tomato plants and gently work it into the soil. This will reduce the tomatoes acid content for sweeter, more delicious tomatoes!"

"Dentures can be cleaned and freshened by soaking in a glass of warm water and 1 tablespoon of baking soda. Let stand undisturbed for 20 – 30 minutes and then rinse clean."

THE VINEGAR BOOK II

This delightful addition to Emily Thacker's series of four books on vinegar takes you through the year, with a vinegar use for each day.

Twelve chapters, one for each month, combine the 365 vinegar based hints with explanations of how vinegar is made, why it is so healthful and how it has been used down through thousands of years.

You will learn of vinegar's uses in cooking and preserving and about its value is preventing diseases. This includes its importance in fighting cancer and arthritis, as well as how vinegar can be used to actually "cook" protein, such as fish.

This book also contains easy directions for making fruit, vegetable and herbal vinegars. You will see how to begin with apple cider vinegar and add rose petals to inspire love and romance, valerian as a sleep aid, bay leaves to sharpen the memory or gota kola to fight stress.

You will also find a recipe for making imitation balsamic vinegar that rivals the expensive varieties for taste and usefulness!

To find out more about *THE VINEGAR BOOK II,* see the publisher's website: http://www.jamesdirect.com or buy it using the order form at the end of this book.

Excerpts from
THE VINEGAR BOOK II

Some of the 365 daily vinegar hints you will find in *THE VINEGAR BOOK II* follow:

Day 70   Vinegar is an antimicrobial agent, effective against yeasts, bacteria and molds.

Day 114   Brown rice vinegar is sweeter that white rice vinegar. This vinegar is used in soy sauces and is good on stir fried foods, especially noodles.

Day 198   Spray greasy pots and pans with a film of full strength white vinegar, let set a few minutes and wash as usual. The grease will wash off easier.

Day 244   Vinegar's acid does more than simply add flavor. It softens tough fibers in food. To make an excellent marinade, begin with 1/2 cup vinegar and 1/2 cup olive oil. Add sliced lemon, bay leaves, thyme, paprika and other spices. Use this to marinate foods before broiling or grilling to shorten cooking time.

Day 238   Fennel vinegar is an excellent topping for broiled fish.

Day 282   Since the 1500s France has been known for truffles pickled in vinegar. Then, they were soaked in hot water and served with butter. This subterranean fungus was thought to be an aphrodisiac.

VINEGAR HOME GUIDE

Distilled or "white" vinegar is usually used for cleaning. Because white vinegar is a colorless liquid it is less likely to discolor articles being cleaned. This guide will show you when to clean with vinegar and when not to clean with vinegar.

Vinegar contains a host of germ fighting components it has both antibiotic and antiseptic properties. It has the ability to actually kill mold and mildew spores. And, it can contain natural tannins which help to preserve foods.

Vinegar is a completely biodegradable product nature can easily break it down into components that feed and nurture plant life. This makes it superior to chemical cleaners that poison the soil today and remain in it and destroy plant life for many years.

This helpful book is packed full of ways to use vinegar around the home, in the garden, on pets and to clean the car, boat or camper. You will want to use vinegar in your humidifier, to strip wallpaper, repair wood scratches kill mold on refrigerator and freezer gaskets and to make both play-clay and mouthwashes.

To find out more about *THE VINEGAR HOME GUIDE,* see the publisher's website: http://www.jamesdirect.com or buy it using the order form at the end of this book.

Excerpts from
VINEGAR HOME GUIDE

"Pure white vinegar makes a great freshener for stale air. Simply use a pump spray to deliver a fine mist to musty areas or to remove cooking or smoking odors. For a fresher scent, use apple cider vinegar."

"A broom with pick up more dust if it is sprayed with vinegar. Just put a cup of warm water in a spray bottle and add a cup of vinegar. Spray the broom before using and occasionally during use."

"Smooth rough hands by dampening them with vinegar, then sprinkling with sugar. Gently rub them together until the sugar melts. Rinse in lukewarm water and pat dry. Hands will be velvet smooth!"

"Improve the flavor of hot dogs by boiling them in water with a dash of vinegar added to it. Pierce them before boiling for less fat (and calories)."

"Keep ants away from plants by making a circle around them with vinegar. Just dribble a generous stream around each plant. It will act as a barrier to wandering ants."

"Control odor on any furry pet by spraying its coat daily with mild vinegar water. A tablespoon in a cup of water is about right for eliminating everyday odors."

"White vinegar can be used to lift coffee and tea stains from clothes. Follow with a soapy washing."

VINEGAR ANNIVERSARY

THE VINEGAR ANNIVERSARY BOOK blends the contents of Emily Thacker's four books on vinegar into one big book!

The original *VINEGAR BOOK* details hundreds of old time healing remedies plus information on how to clean with vinegar. You will learn about the many different kinds of vinegar – from apple cider, wine, rice and malt to more exotic kinds such as banana and date.

THE VINEGAR BOOK II offers 365 vinegar uses to let you try a new one every day of the year.

THE VINEGAR HOME GUIDE focuses on using vinegar for cleaning and disinfecting around the home, yard and garden.

THE VINEGAR DIET BOOK brings all the healthy goodness of vinegar to the table in an exciting, safe way to easily control weight. This remarkable way to manage weight offers wholesome, nourishing insight into managing what you eat. You will find this is the easiest, most foolproof diet plan you have ever tried!

To find out more about *THE VINEGAR ANNIVERSARY BOOK,* see the publisher's website: http://www.jamesdirect.com or buy it using the order form at the end of this book.

Excerpts from
VINEGAR ANNIVERSARY

"Vinegar is part of a healthy diet and has been used for centuries to aid health. Scientists tell us vinegar was probably part of the primordial soup of life. It is needed to burn fats and carbohydrates. The acid we know as vinegar is also used by the body as an aid in neutralizing poisons."

"Fortified vinegars contain fruits and vegetables, blended with vinegar, to form toppings and sauces. Recipes for several diet fortifying vinegars can be found in this book."

"Banish foot odor by soaking feet in strong tea. Follow with a rinse made from a cup of warm water and a cup of apple cider vinegar."

"Old times have long recommended taking a teaspoon of apple cider vinegar, every day, in a tall glass of water."

"As little as one tablespoon of vinegar per quart of water can make a difference in the calcium that is pulled from boiled soup bones."

"Vinegar, added to fish dishes, helps to eliminate the traditional fishy odor. It also helps get rid of fish smells at clean up time."

"Soak fresh vegetables in water with a little vinegar added to it to rid them of garden bugs."

EMILY'S DISASTER GUIDE OF NATURAL REMEDIES

EMILY'S NEW GUIDE TO NATURAL TREATMENTS FOR INFECTIOUS DISEASE

Our world is changing. Like it or not, in our post-September 11 world, we live under the threat of a terrorist strike.

Hurricane Katrina has reminded us that nature can be brutal, with heavy consequences for those in nature's path or for citizens unprepared.

Our increased mobility with air transportation means any disease outbreak, anywhere in the world, can be at our doorstep in mere days.

EMILY'S DISASTER GUIDE OF NATURAL REMEDIES is a unique guide written to highlight some of the many threats we face, both natural and manmade, and ways to prepare and protect your family.

Included in this guide is an overview of current events and the state our communities are in. You will also find a list of infectious diseases and conditions, along with possible treatments.

PLUS each book contains its own Emergency Preparedness Checklist and Emergency Family Plan to help your family prepare for any emergency.

To find out more about *EMILY'S DISASTER GUIDE OF NATURAL REMEDIES,* see the publisher's website: http://www.jamesdirect.com or buy it using the order form at the end of this book.

Excerpts from
EMILY'S DISASTER GUIDE OF NATURAL REMEDIES

EMILY'S NEW GUIDE TO NATURAL TREATMENTS FOR INFECTIOUS DISEASE

"It doesn't take the actions of a terrorist or a new strain of an old virus to have a devastating impact on our lives. Sometimes, the event comes naturally.

August 2005 saw Hurricane Katrina slam into the gulf coast states with ferocious intensity. While the news that more than 1,800 people lost their lives was the obvious headline of that tragic event, there was another untold story that we can learn from. More than 80% of New Orleans was flooded, and the flood waters themselves lingered for weeks. In those flood waters grew bacteria. Toxic chemicals, raw sewage and bacteria invaded homes and drinking supplies sickening scores more. It was reported that several people died of dehydration due to a lack of clean drinking water because of contamination."

"An emergency readiness kit may be one of the most important preparations you can make. It could be the difference between safety and security and being a victim of circumstances."

"Fevers are greatly reduced when treated with willow tea in copious amounts."

"Vinegar can attack can attack and kill harmful bacteria that has entered the digestive tract. This may lessen the likelihood of the body developing toxemia and other blood-borne infections."

THE HYDROGEN PEROXIDE BOOK

One of the most unusual books I have written, because it not only covers the healthy attributes of hydrogen peroxide but also talks about its use as an alternate fuel source. In these times of concern about running out of complex petroleum based fuels, hydrogen peroxide's simple formula and renewable attributes make it an important part of both today's energy production and tomorrow's energy needs.

In addition to being an excellent propellant, hydrogen peroxide has a long history of medicinal use. It is well know for its ability to cleanse and disinfect wounds. Less well known is its ability to disinfect water and sanitize many kinds of medical equipment.

Hydrogen peroxide is used to dissolve earwax and to prevent infection in scrapes and cuts. It is also part of some enjoyable, but safe, chemical experiments for children.

To buy an additional copy of *THE HYDROGEN PEROXIDE BOOK*, see the publisher's website: http://www.jamesdirect.com or use the order form at the end of this book.

EXCERPTS FROM
THE HYDROGEN PEROXIDE BOOK

"The United States Department of Housing and Urban Development includes hydrogen peroxide on their list of approved disinfectants for 'certain biohazards.' This list includes treatment for ridding homes of certain molds that are hazardous to the health of any inhabitants."

"Take a mouthful of hydrogen peroxide and rinse it around your teeth and gums to help keep your mouth fresh, clean and free of germs."

"To rid hands of both germs and strong odors, wash with a mixture of hydrogen peroxide and baking soda."

"Make your own whitening toothpaste using hydrogen peroxide. Mix small amounts of hydrogen peroxide and baking soda until it forms a soft paste. Brush twice a day with whitening paste, being careful not to swallow any of the solution. Rinse."

"You can also use an eyebrow brush to apply peroxide to brows you wish to lighten. Be careful not to apply to skin area around brows, as skin may also lighten."

"Add a few tablespoons of hydrogen peroxide to your electric dishwasher detergent for greater cleaning and disinfecting strength."

Thank You!

Thank you, once again, dear reader, for your continued interest in natural healing ways. It has been a pleasure to bring you this book, and all its exciting uses for honey.

If you have a natural healing remedy, unique or special cleaning method or fun, old-time recipe that your family has used, would you consider sharing it with other readers just like yourself? If I use it in one of my upcoming books, you will receive a free copy of the book upon printing.

Please fill out the form that follow and mail it back to me. If the form is missing or isn't available, feel free to use a sheet of paper and mail your ideas in to us.

Thank you again, and my warmest wishes for a long, healthy, happy life.

Emily Thacker

Emily, here is one of my favorite uses for honey:

_____

_____

_____

_____

_____

_____

Can we use your name and city when crediting this remedy in the book?

❑ Yes, please credit this remedy to:

_____

❑ No, please use my remedy, but do not use my name in the book.

Either way, yes or no, if I use your remedy, I'll send you a free copy of the new edition of home remedies.

Your remedy can be one which uses honey, or simply one that you feel others would like to know about.

My favorite chapter in *"The Honey Book"* is:

_____

_____

The most helpful remedy I appreciated in *"The Honey Book"* is:

_____

_____

_____

_____

_____

_____

What I liked best about *"The Honey Book"* is:

_____

_____

_____

_____

_____

_____

_____

_____

Would you be interested in hearing about my new
cookbook when it becomes available?

_____

My name and mailing address is:

_____

_____

_____

If you have any comments or experiences to add to the
information you've read in this collection, or if you have
information for subsequent editions, please address your letters
to:

Emily Thacker
PO Box 980
Hartville, OH 44632

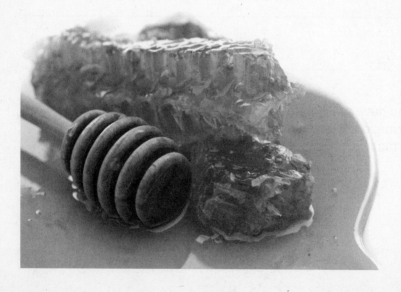

✂ please cut here

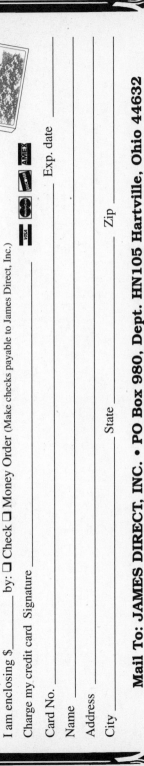

The Honey Book

90-DAY MONEY-BACK GUARANTEE

☐ **YES!** Please rush _____ additional copies of The Honey Book and my FREE copy of the bonus booklet *"Arthritis Remedies & Folklore"* for only $19.95 plus $3.98 postage & handling. I understand that I must be completely satisfied or I can return it within 90 days for a full and prompt refund of my purchase price. The FREE gift is mine to keep regardless. *Want to save even more?* Do a favor for a close relative or friend and order two books for only $30 postpaid.

I am enclosing $ _____ by: ☐ Check ☐ Money Order (Make checks payable to James Direct, Inc.)

Charge my credit card   Signature _____

Card No. _____   Exp. date _____

Name _____

Address _____

City _____ State _____ Zip _____

Mail To: JAMES DIRECT, INC. • PO Box 980, Dept. HN105 Hartville, Ohio 44632

http://www.jamesdirect.com

✂ please cut here -------------------------------------

Use this coupon to order "The Honey Book" for a friend or family member -- or copy the ordering information onto a plain piece of paper and mail to:

The Honey Book
Dept. HN105
PO Box 980
Hartville, Ohio 44632

Preferred Customer Reorder Form

Order this...	If you want a book on...	Cost...	Number of Copies...
Garlic: Nature's Natural Companion	Exciting scientific research on garlic's ability to promote good health. Find out for yourself why garlic has the reputation of being able to heal almost magically! Newest in Emily's series of natural heath books!	$9.95	
Amish Gardening Secrets	You too can learn the special gardening secrets the Amish use to produce huge tomato plants and bountiful harvests. Information packed 800-plus collection for you to tinker with and enjoy.	$9.95	
The Vinegar Home Guide	Learn how to clean and freshen with natural, environmentally-safe vinegar in the house, garden and laundry. Plus, delicious home-style recipes!	$9.95	
Emily's Disaster Guide of Natural Remedies	Emily's new guide to infectious diseases & their threat on our health. What happens if we can't get to the pharmacy – or the shelves are empty, *what then?* What if the electricity goes out – and stays out? What if my neighborhood was quarantined? How would I feed my family? Handle first aid? 208 page book!	$9.95	

Any combination of the above $9.95 items qualifies for the following discounts...

	Total NUMBER of $9.95 items	

Order any 2 items for: $15.95

Order any 4 items for: $24.95

Order any 6 items for: $34.95 and receive 7th item FREE

Any additional items for: $5 each

Order any 3 items for: $19.95

Order any 5 items for: $29.95

FEATURED SELECTIONS

	Total COST of $9.95 items	

		Cost	Copies
The Vinegar Anniversary Book	Completely updated with the latest research and brand new remedies and uses for apple cider vinegar. Handsome coffee table collector's edition you'll be proud to display. ***Big 208-page book!***	$12.95	
The Magic of Baking Soda	*Plain Old Baking Soda A Drugstore in A Box?* Doctors & researchers have discovered baking soda has amazing healing properties! Over 600 health & Household Hints. *Great Recipes Too!*	$12.95	
The Honey Book	Amazing Honey Remedies to relieve arthritis pain, kill germs, heal infection and much more!	$19.95	
The Magic of Hydrogen Peroxide	An Ounce of Hydrogen Peroxide is worth a Pound of Cure! Hundreds of health cures, household uses & home remedy uses for hydrogen peroxide contained in this breakthrough volume.	$19.95	
Vinegar Formula Guide	This one-of-a-kind, ground breaking book gives you exact formulas and measurements for ALL of your vinegar applications! In it you'll find step-by-step, easy-to-use instructions for home health remedies, cleaning projects and more!	$19.95	

Order any 2 or more Featured Selections for only $10 each...

Postage & Handling	$3.98*
TOTAL	

90-Day Money-Back Guarantee

*** Shipping of 10 or more books = $6.96**

Please rush me the items marked above. I understand that I must be completely satisfied or I can return any item within 90 days with proof of purchase for a full and prompt refund of my purchase price.

I am enclosing $_____ by: ❏ Check ❏ Money Order (Make checks payable to James Direct Inc)

Charge my credit card Signature _____

Card No. _____ Exp. Date _____

Name _____ Address _____

City _____ State_____ Zip _____

Telephone Number (_____) _____

❏ Yes! I'd like to know about freebies, specials and new products before they are nationally advertised. My email address is: _____

Mail To: **James Direct Inc.** • PO Box 980, Dept. A1342 • Hartville, Ohio 44632
Customer Service (330) 877-0800 • *http://www.jamesdirect.com*

©2014 JDI A223IM

GARLIC: NATURE'S NATURAL COMPANION

Explore the very latest studies and new remedies using garlic to help with cholesterol, blood pressure, asthma, arthritis, digestive disorders, bacteria, cold and flu symptoms, and MUCH MORE! Amazing cancer studies!

AMISH GARDENING SECRETS

There's something for everyone in *Amish Gardening Secrets.* This BIG collection contains over 800 gardening hints, suggestions, time savers and tonics that have been passed down over the years in Amish communities and elsewhere.

THE VINEGAR HOME GUIDE

Emily Thacker presents her second volume of hundreds of all-new vinegar tips. Use versatile vinegar to add a low-sodium zap of flavor to your cooking, as well as getting your house "white-glove" clean for just pennies. Plus, safe and easy tips on shining and polishing brass, copper & pewter and removing stubborn stains & static cling in your laundry!

EMILY'S DISASTER GUIDE OF NATURAL REMEDIES

Emily's most important book yet! If large groups of the population become sick at the same time, the medical services in this country will become stressed to capacity. *What then?* We will all need to know what to do! Over 307 natural cures, preventatives, cure-alls and ways to prepare to naturally treat & prevent infectious disease.

THE VINEGAR ANNIVERSARY BOOK

Handsome coffee table edition and brand new information on Mother Nature's Secret Weapon – apple cider vinegar!

THE MAGIC OF BAKING SODA

We all know baking soda works like magic around the house. It cleans, deodorizes & works wonders in the kitchen and in the garden. But did you know it's an effective remedy for allergies, bladder infection, heart disorders… *and MORE!*

THE HONEY BOOK

Each page is packed with healing home remedies and ways to use honey to heal wounds, fight tooth decay, treat burns, fight fatigue, restore energy, ease coughs and even make cancer-fighting drugs more effective. Great recipes too!

THE MAGIC OF HYDROGEN PEROXIDE

Hundreds of health cures & home remedy uses for hydrogen peroxide. You'll be amazed to see how a little hydrogen peroxide mixed with a pinch of this or that from your cupboard can do everything from relieving chronic pain to making age spots go away! Easy household cleaning formulas too!

VINEGAR FORMULA GUIDE

Studies have shown vinegar to be effective at not only cleaning and disinfecting, but also as a natural home remedy for conditions such as lowering cholesterol, fighting disease, easing arthritis, improving circulation and more! Now learn the exact formulas and measurements for EACH home remedy and cleaning project in a concise, easy-to-read format! No more guesswork!

* Each Book has its own FREE Bonus!